# Alkaline Diet Cookbook

**Lose Weight Quickly and Permanently, Reset and Cleanse Your Body with More than 100 Plant-Based Recipes for Beginners.**

**Plan to Balance Your pH, Be More Energetic, and Prevent Degenerative Diseases.**

**A Natural Approach to Dieting Guide to Detox the Liver & amp; Regain total Health.**

**Author: James Linner**

# Table of Content

# Introduction

Are you curious about the widely followed Alkaline Diet? Have you heard people sharing their improved health experience after just the three weeks of an alkaline diet? Are you wondering what makes this diet different from the rest? Well, this cookbook is all about the alkaline diet, how it works, what benefits it promises, and what a person can consume on this diet. All the 14 chapters in this book discuss the basics of the alkaline, and there is a complete section of recipes providing a range of flavors, all the essential nutrients in a variety of styles. If you are looking for a healthy yet delicious diet, then this cookbook can provide you all, from breakfast meals to lunch, dinner, desserts, soups, salad, snacks and smoothies, you can practically find any of your favorite meals, designed keeping the alkaline approach in consideration. Quick and easy to cook recipes are all that make this cookbook a must-read. Learn more about the alkaline diet and experience all its claimed health benefits.

# Chapter 1: Alkaline Diet Basics

## What is Alkaline Diet:

In the 1800s, and ash centric dietary approach was discovered, and it led to a better understanding of the acidic and alkaline-forming food. This approach says that when the food is processed, digested, and assimilated; it releases either acid or alkaline "ash" as a final product in the body. This metabolic waste can then directly affect the acidity or alkalinity of the body. This dietary approach suggests that eating more of such food that will leave more alkaline products in the body, thus maintaining its alkalinity. Whereas those with acidic nature will only leave acidic by-products, including toxins that are hazardous for human health.

All vegetables, fruits, nuts, and legumes are categorized as the alkaline group, whereas eggs, grains, meat, sugars, dairy, and alcohols, etc. are present in the Acidic group and the rest of the food can be termed as neutral. The acidity and alkalinity of a substance are calculated by the pH levels or the number of hydrogen ions in that substance. The pH scale rates any substances between 0-14 to represent its acidic or alkaline nature. Acids have values from 0-6, whereas 7 is for neutrality, and 7 to 14 values are for alkaline substances.

The internal pH levels of our body are also fixed, in most of the organs there are alkaline conditions, and whereas in some others, like stomach, it gets acidic. Internal pH values indicate the optimal condition required for the functioning of each organ. A pH of 2 or 3.5 in the stomach is essential for the digestive enzymes to work on the proteins, but it the food should be alkaline to be processed in the small intestine; that is why pancreatic and hepatic enzymes are added to increase the pH value of the food. Human blood is also alkaline in nature, having a pH of 7.44 to 7.36 on the pH scale. All the hormones or blood components can function best at this pH. If the acidic metabolic waste enters into our blood, it automatically disrupts the optimal pH level. Resultantly, the body tends to respond negatively to this change. The disruption of pH levels also affects the kidneys function, and it was be assessed by checking the increased acidity of the urine sample.

## The Science Behind Alkaline Diet:

The science behind the alkaline diet is that it consists of all of the ingredients that are digested to produce alkaline metabolic ash. Once we consumed food, it goes through a series of the digestive process; the food passes through changing pH environments and finally breaks down into usable energy units. Most of the enzymes in our digestive system, except for the stomach, require alkaline and or neutral environment to work on food molecules. Unavailability of such food can cause indigestion, the death of many gut microbes, and inhibit the absorption of a number of nutrients. The alkaline diet neutralizes the gastric juices and helps in better digestion throughout the gut.

The idea of the alkaline surfaced with the observation of some experts claiming certain food items as more acid-forming than the other. These food items release more calcium from the bones and end up causing osteoporosis in early age. Further studies then later revealed that it is not just a few items, rather a number of items having low pH, which are linked to diseases like bone weakness, cancer, heart strokes, gut ailments, diabetes, bloating, headaches, etc.

## Benefits of Using the Alkaline Diet:

The following are proved to be the scientifically proven health benefits of the alkaline diet, which has been commonly reported by many of the alkaline diet followers.

**1.    Weight loss**

There are many diet plans which may promise weight loss, but the means of achieving that aim may sometime sound impractical; however, that's not the case of the alkaline diet. This meal plan works through slow and progressive bodily changes; it leads to an optimum internal body condition which supports high metabolic rates, improved digestion, and better absorption of the nutrients. The diet is also limiting the consumption of animal or saturated fat. Consequently, it contributes to weight loss, and a person may lose 2-3 pounds of weight within a month, given that he follows the diet according to the set limits and restriction.

## 2.    Better kidney health

The health of the kidney depends upon the concentration on the purity of the blood. If there are lots of toxins or other excretory products in the blood, kidneys would need to work with extra strain to purify the blood. A toxic and saturated internal environment with low pH can lead to kidney damages or other obstructions in the kidney functions. According to a 2017 study, people with a more acidic diet showed clear symptoms of kidney damage at some level than those who were on an alkaline diet. By minimizing the intake of acidic proteins helped to improve the kidney condition.

## 3.    Reduces the Risk of Cancer

Experts believe that alkaline can also help in the treatment of cancer and consider that this diet also supports healthy body cells during chemotherapy. Though there are no proven medical evidence or studies conducted that could directly link the approach to the treatment of cancer, but when people with such a health condition were given an alkaline diet, they showed clear symptoms of improvement. European Prospective Investigation into Cancer and Nutrition, EPICN says that a diet rich in vitamins A, C, and fiber greatly helps in reducing the risks of cancer, and an alkaline diet is full of such ingredients.  And the American Cancer Society has also prescribed a diet to alkaline diet to fight the negative effects of cancer. The society has warned against the use of soft drinks, processed foods, and high-fat products, and recommended a diet rich in fruit, whole grains, and vegetables.

## 4.      Prevents Cardiac diseases

A poor diet rich in bad cholesterol and saturated fat, along with low activity, is the major cause of cardiac diseases these days. A diet consisting of saturated fat leads to higher blood cholesterols and resultantly leads to high blood pressure and, eventually, cardiac strokes. The alkaline diet also boosts the production of growth hormone in the body, which sparks the rate of metabolism in the body. It improves the heart's condition and its functioning. An alkaline diet also restricts the caloric and fat intake, which is ideal for all the cardiac patients. Red meat like lamb, beef, or pork, are also prohibited in this diet.

## 5.      Improved Growth:

Hormones act as a catalyst of change and function in our body. None of the metabolic activity can be carried without the release of some type of hormone. Alkaline diet help in the improved production of the hormones, especially the growth hormones.

The hormones increase the brain's functionality and enhance memory. Overall a person feels healthier and more live. Experts believe that an alkaline diet provides the necessary conditions to the hormone-producing cells for the production of those growth hormones.

## 6.    Treats Back Pain

We cannot say with certainty how the diet actually treats back pain, but the increased intake of minerals in this diet can be the contributing factor of reducing the backache. The diet can only work gradually along with the necessary medical treatment, not in entirety.

## 7.    Prevents Osteoporosis:

It is a condition in which bones get weak due to the lack of absorption of calcium or loss of calcium from the bones. In this condition, the calcium is lost from the body through urine. Some cases suggested that the alkaline diet can help in reducing the loss of calcium from the body, thus retain the bones' strength and shape. As the person take more vegetables and fruits in his diet, and less of the processed products, his bones grow and repair naturally. The diet can not completely prevent the disease but can definitely help in containing the condition.

## 8. Healthy Muscles:

With age, the muscles can lose their mass, strength, and form, which could result in more falls and bone fractures. Pain and weakness are two obvious results. A recent study conducted in 2013 suggested that the alkaline diet can help in improving muscle health. In another twin study, the researchers studied 2689 females with muscle weakness and discovered that there was a significant improvement in muscle health of all the participants who followed the alkaline diet.

## 9. Arthritis:

It's a bone-related disorder where the lack of calcium and other mineral leads to the degeneration of bone cartilages and coverings. This results in pain and swelling in the joints and immobility of the bones. The alkaline diet stops the release of excessive calcium in the body as it neutralizes the effects of acid produced. Thus, helping to improve the bone structure and makes them stronger.

## 10. Insomnia:

Most of the oxidants and toxins produced inside the body are acidic radicals which damage the brain cells, neurotransmitters, and the whole sleep cycle of a person. Alkaline food neutralizes those toxins and the blood, which cures insomnia to some extent.

## 11. Gout:

Gout is that disease which is caused by the accumulation of uric acid in the body. Alkaline food can help reduce the level of uric acid and can prevent gout threats. It is safe to switch to an alkaline diet, especially when you want to avoid medications.

# Chapter 2: How does Alkaline Diet Work?

Food that is capable of producing acidic metabolic waste in the body is considered as acid-forming food. Some complex proteins, processed food items, saturated fats, sugars, beverages, etc. are all acidic in this regard. It is discovered that by omitting all such acidic ingredients from the diet and adding more of the food items, that can produce alkaline waste, to the meal can help improve human health. The diet itself does not change the pH of the blood and the body, but it does affect the pH of saliva, kidneys, and the entire digestive system, which indirectly affects the rest of the body. Thus, alkaline food helps in better working of the digestive system, optimal absorption of nutrients, and ensures prevention from acidic and harmful toxins.

In order to analyze the acid load human body can bear, Manz and Remez had also created a scale named "Potential Renal Acid load," also known as the PRAL scale. On this scale, 0 is for neutrality, a negative value means alkalinity, and a positive value means that the substance is acidic. Meat, cheese, sugar, grain, etc. all show higher PRAL values on this scale, which means these food items are more acidic in nature and produce acidic ash after digestion. On the other hand, fruits and vegetables give a negative value on the PRAL scale and thus recognized as alkaline-forming.

## Understanding pH

To explain in simple words, pH indicates the level of acidity of a substance. The lower the pH values, the higher the acidity is. The entire pH scale ranges from 1 to 14 in values. Substances with pH values lower than 6 are termed as acidic. PH 7 indicates neutrality, and any value higher than this is termed as alkaline. The greater the value, the more alkaline the substance is.

The food we eat also varies in its pH value; some substances are rich in acids, whereas others are more alkaline. There are no marked categories to distinguish a pure alkaline diet from a non-alkaline one, except to identify the items with low pH and avoid them. Items like lemons, oranges, meat, dairy, and processed food, all are acidic in nature.

## Ways to Follow Alkaline Diet:

Unlike other health-oriented diets, the Alkaline diet takes a different approach; it puts no limit to the portion size or caloric intake, rather it restricts any food that is acid-forming. That aim must be kept in mind before starting out on this dietary plan.

### 1.  Starting from Scratch:

Most of the food that we eat daily is alkaline-forming mixed with some proportion of acid-forming food. To start on this diet, learn about the food you are consuming and identify it as being acid or alkaline-forming.  Learn more about the recipes that make good use of alkaline food. Then prepare yourself for the much-needed lifestyle changes.

### 2.  Eat and Drink Alkaline Forming Food:

Health experts believe that through healthy food and drinks termed as alkaline-forming, one can maintain the natural alkalinity of the body. The aim is to reduce the daily acid load through food that could counter and neutralize the effect. Meat, dairy, sugars, and refined carbs are capable of releasing acidic by-products in the body, so these items should be avoided and replaced with more fruits and vegetables. Remember, not to confuse an alkaline diet with the acid reflux diet; both are completely different approaches; the former restricts the acid-forming food, whereas the latter restricts the consumption of food that could trigger acidity in the stomach.

### 3. The 80/20 Rule:

This rule best describes the alkaline diet and lays out a complete plan of adoption. It is true that when it comes to food, one cannot abstain completely from certain food that is labeled as acid-forming. Maintain complete alkalinity of the diet is next to impossible. Therefore, this 80/20 rule provides a perfect window for all such errors. It means that 80 percent of the meal should be alkaline-forming, and the rest of the 20 percent can be acid-forming. This 80/20 rule has emerged from repeated tests and experiments, and it was found to be most effective for everyone irrespective of age, gender, and health conditions.

### 4. Go Organic and Go Green!

Normally there is one fit formula that could instantly tell you what to eat and not to eat on an alkaline diet. But there is one standard criterion that works for almost every healthy diet is to eat organic fruits and vegetables. That same mantra also works well for the alkaline diet. Whenever you feel confused about this diet, simply add more fruits and vegetables, especially green ones.

Today when we hit the grocery store, we find tons of processed food products, though such items promise convenience and ease; they are filled with fine carbs, preservatives, sugars, and other acid-forming substances. Almost 90 percent of such store packed items are acidic. Therefore, they should be avoided and replaced with more organic ingredients. Plant-based items, in this regard, are the safest option to go for.

## 5. Hydration

Whenever you switch to a health-oriented diet plan, the body gradually goes into a transition state. It leads to more dehydration and loss of water. Hydration is important all the time, as it supports the metabolism. But it becomes even more important when the metabolism is taking a turn. Water itself is a neutralizer, so the more you consume water, the more it will neutralize the acidic pH of the water. However, for the alkaline diet, the water can be filtered then be turned into alkaline water with pH 9.5. According to the thumb rule, a person should drink water 6 to 18 cups of water per day.

## 6. Slow Transition

Since we are not habitual of consuming alkaline-forming food all the time. A sudden transition may not support the existing metabolic rate. It is not a matter of days, but it takes 1 week to detoxify the body and allow it to adapt to the change. Don't think of its as a diet; take it as a lifestyle approach that requires gradual changes.

## 7. Use Supplements:

Food alone sometimes falls short of the much-needed alkalinity to balance out the internal pH of the body, so experts prescribe certain supplements that help in the transition process. The supplements that are recommended for the alkaline diet includes green powders that are extracted from plant-based sources. Then there is alkalinizing water, which is made by using a water ionizer. Certain minerals are also termed as a buffer to acids in the body; they mainly include calcium, potassium, magnesium, and sodium. To meet the needs of omega 3 and omega 6, the dieter can switch to omega supplements, which are available in a wide variety.

## Pre-Diet Detoxification:

Like every other health-oriented, alkaline approach also require a pre-diet preparation. Since we constantly consume acid-forming food items, it tends to build up an Acid load in the body. It needs one week of detoxification for the body to get rid off this acid load. In order to shake off the unhealthy dietary habits, it is important to cleanse the body of the oxidants and toxins, then take a fresh start:

1. Nothing works better than fresh salads when you want to cleanse your body. Salads contain all the ingredients that are most suitable to the alkaline diet, all the green leafy vegetables, juicy sprouts, green beans, asparagus, etc.; moreover, you don't need much of the ingredients to add flavor to the salad. A drizzle of olive oil, apple cider, and crushed peppers can make it all delicious.

2.  Increase the intake of vegetables in your diet by adding them as a side meal to every entrée. Steam and roasted vegetables are the right choices for alkaline dieters; without drastically increasing the caloric intake, you can add essential nutrients, vitamins, and fibers to the table. Vegetables contain a variety of phytonutrients that work as natural detoxifiers.

3.  Another great way to detoxify the body in a short period of time is to add fruits and vegetable juices to the basic diet. Instead of having fried or bake snacks, start taking fresh juices in between the meals. Juices are also a good way to fight the cravings. Take a glass of mixed juices at least one or three times a day. Spinach, parsley, cabbage, and carrot juice are great for the early detoxification.

4.  Fruits provide a natural and organic substitute to table sugar. By adding more fruits to the diet, you limit the intake of other processed sugars and carbs. Add them to the smoothies and salads.

5.  There is yet another way to get rid of all the toxins, and that is to add herbal teas to the diet. Dandelion, chamomile, sage, or nettle tea are a few refreshing options to go for.

# The First Week of Alkaline Diet:

It is usually the first week of the diet that is more crucial. In this week, a dieter starts to experience mild discomfort due to the nature of the changes the body goes through. The withdrawal effects are always there whether you stop consuming anything; the body is habitual of consuming. The same is the case with the alkaline diet. Sugar, salt, and meat are three major ingredients that everyone consumes in a normal routine since these ingredients are restricted on the alkaline diet; the dieter will feel natural cravings for these food items.

The first two days of the alkaline diet might not feel like much. Most dieters do not experience any change at all during the first two days. During this time, the acid load remains almost the same. But as time goes on, the dieter starts feeling more dehydrated and drained. This change is normal and common to all. Some people may experience lethargy and lower energy levels. But with scheduled meals and constant intake of water or juices, these effects can be controlled. The third and fourth days are considered the hardest, and the dieter may get constant cravings to eat sugary food and lots of meat. The transition remains easier for vegetarians, as they already don't feel the urge to eat meat.

A person can easily fight those craving by frequently consuming small low caloric meals and juices. Fresh fruits, mixed juices, and vegetables are a good way to satisfy your cravings. When a person passes through this stage, the body starts embracing the change, and by the end of the fifth day of the week, the acid load reduces to a minimum level. The dieter feels fresh and light. Though he may experience some cravings, that changes by the end of the sixth day. By the end of the week, the metabolic rates auto-adjust to the new diet, and the dieter feels more active and healthier.

## Alkaline Testing:

The change in the alkalinity of the body cannot be identified through visible symptoms. It has to be checked through certain tests. The best and easy way is to test the pH of the blood, urine, and saliva. Compare their pH values with the optimal pH levels and analyze if you need to decrease the Acidic load of the body.

1.  **Blood pH:**

The normal pH of blood varies for 7.35 to 7.45 pH on the scale. It means that the human body is naturally slightly alkaline in nature. When this value decreases even in a small amount, the enzymic activity and the flow of the essential hormones and cells are disturbed or disrupted. The blood pH changes when there is a toxic buildup of metabolic waste.

2.  **Urine pH**

In response to the increased Acid Load in the body, kidneys function excessively to regain the alkalinity of the blood. In this process, more of the uric acid and other acid byproducts are released through the Urine. A consistently low pH value of the urine, therefore, indicates that the body is suffering from an acidic build-up. The normal pH of urine ranges from 6 to 7.5, so it is slightly acidic to neutral and neutral to the slightly basic in nature.

### 3. Saliva pH:

Digestion starts right from the mouth, mainly because of the saliva and its enzymes. The enzymes in saliva can function best at 5.6 to 7.9 pH. Saliva's pH is another determinant of the body's pH condition. And it can be tested to do the same.

### Testing Urine and Saliva pH

Saliva pH testing strips are available both online and in the market, which can instantly indicate the pH level of both the saliva and the urine. Both can be tested through different procedures.

### 1. Urine test:

Test the pH of urine in the morning before eating or drinking anything; in this way, you will avoid all other intervening variables from the test. Wet the pH test strips with the urine sample for 2 seconds and then match the color that appears on the strip with the given labels on the box and identify if it is equal to the normal pH of urine or not.

## 2. Saliva Test:

A saliva test is another easy test that any individual can carry out at home with the use of easily available saliva pH testing strips. Never put the whole strip directly into the mouth to check the pH. But slightly dap the strip with some saliva sample and leave it for 2 seconds until the color appears on the strip. Then match the color with those given on the table. Remember not to test the saliva's pH directly after eating or drinking anything. Wait for 30 minutes and then check the pH of your saliva.

# Chapter 3: Learning About Alkaline Diet

Not every food is an alkaline food, and not every food that we eat is metabolized into alkaline ash. It is imperative to look for substances that can give non-acidic metabolic waste. For an alkaline diet, some dietary changes are required and need to be adopted. Moreover, it needs a concerted effort to maintain the intake of alkalinizing food like as follows:

## What is Alkaline Water?

The drinking water that we regularly consume has a pH level of 7, which is considered neutral. Whereas water, having a higher pH value than 7 is classified as the Alkaline Water. It usually has a pH value of 8 to 9.5. Since the acid-forming food has become an integral part of our lives, alkaline water is needed along with alkaline food to counter the effects of such toxic diet. It has been brought into use for its following health benefits:

- Weight loss
- Strengthens the immune system
- Prevention of cancer
- Detoxification
- Anti-aging effects

# Alkalinizing Food

Remember that the alkaline diet does not mean to take only food that has a high pH value. It's not merely the nature and chemical composition of the food that matters here, but what is really important to understand is that what type of metabolic waste is produced from the food. If it is produced alkaline waste after digestion, that means that such food is good to consume. Based on this approach, we can identify several food items as being alkalinizing or alkaline-forming.

1. Potatoes
2. Peas
3. Fruit juices
4. Vegetable juices
5. Plain yogurt
6. Beans like lima, soy, green, and snap
7. Arrowroot flour
8. Herbal teas
9. Sprouted seeds of alfalfa, radish, and chia
10. Whey
11. Unsprouted sesame
12. Nuts like almonds, fresh coconut, and chestnuts
13. Fresh unsalted butter
14. Garlic

15.    Cayenne pepper

16.    Gelatin

17.    Most herbs

18.    Miso

19.    Vegetable and sea salt

20.    All spices

21.    Vanilla extract

22.    Sweeteners like raw, unpasteurized honey, brown rice
       syrup

23.    Brewer's yeast

## Acid Forming Food

As per definition, any food item when metabolized produces
acidic metabolic waste is known as acid-forming food. Such food
is not recommended on the alkaline diet. Remember, there is a
significant difference between Acidic food and Acid Forming
food, the former is the food which is acidic in nature, whereas the
latter is capable of producing acidic by-products. Lemon juice is
acidic in nature, but it is not termed as Acid forming; rather, it
has alkalizing effects. Here is a brief list of the items that are
considered acid-forming.

1.    All meat: beef, pork, lamb, fish, and chicken

2.    Rice: white, brown, or basmati

3.      Cornmeal, rye

4.      Popcorn

5.      Pasta

6.      Cheese

7.      Wheat germ

8.      Colas

9.      Alcoholic drinks

10.     Grains such as millet, flax, quinoa, and amaranth

11.     Coffee and caffeinated drinks

12.     Ketchup

13.     Mayonnaise

14.     Sweetened yogurt

15.     Refined table salt

16.     Soy sauce

17.     Nutmeg

18.     Mustard

19.     White vinegar

20.     Tobacco

## What to Enjoy

**THE PRAL Standard:** Although we have extensively discussed the acid-forming and alkaline-forming food along with their suitability to the alkaline diet when it comes to grocery shopping, it is the PRAL value that is used as a standard to check if the food is suitable to the alkaline diet. In general, all the alkalinizing food are good for this diet, and according to the Potential renal acid load formula, given by Thomas Remer, food with negative PRAL value are most suitable for this diet. According to this formula and the PRAL table, the following ingredients are good to eat on an Alkaline diet.

- Fruits
- Vegetables
- Plants based oils
- Plant milk: Soy, Almond, Coconut, or Hemp milk
- Nuts
- Seeds
- Nondairy egg substitutes

| FOOD | Potential Renal Acid Load (PRAL) mEq/100g |
|---|---|
| **Fruit** | |
| Apples | -2.2 |
| Lemon juice | -2.5 |
| Apricots | -4.8 |
| Oranges | -2.7 |
| Black Currants | -6.5 |
| Peaches | -2.4 |
| Pears | -2.9 |

| | |
|---|---|
| Raisins | -2.1 |
| Strawberries | -2.2 |
| Watermelon | -1.9 |
| **Vegetables** | |
| Carrots | -4.9 |
| Celery | -5.2 |
| Lettuce | -2.5 |
| Broccoli | -1.2 |
| Asparagus | -0.4 |
| Cucumber | -0.8 |
| Green beans | -3.1 |
| Potatoes | -4.0 |
| Spinach | -14.0 |
| Tomatoes | -3.1 |
| **Condiments and Sweets** | |
| Honey | -0.3 |
| **Beverages** | |
| Coffee | -1.4 |
| Red wine | -2.4 |
| White wine | -1.2 |
| Apple juice, unsweetened | -2.2 |
| Orange juice, unsweetened | -2.9 |

| Lemon juice, unsweetened | -2.5 |
| --- | --- |

## What to Avoid

The PRAL formula and criterion avoid all such errors that make people confuse an alkaline diet with an acid reflux diet. The food that should be avoided on this diet shows a positive PRAL value, which means that they tend to increase the Acid Load of the body. According to these values, the following major ingredients should be avoided on this diet:

- Meat
- Poultry
- Fish
- Dairy
- Eggs
- Grain

| Acidic Foods | |
| --- | --- |
| **FOOD** | **Potential Renal Acid Load mEq/100g** |
| **Meat** | |
| Chicken | 8.7 |
| Turkey | 9.9 |
| Beef | 7.8 |
| Pork | 7.9 |
| Salami | 11.6 |
| | |
| **Milk, Dairy, and Eggs** | |
| | |
| Cottage cheese, plain | 8.7 |
| Cheddar cheese | 26.4 |
| Egg white | 1.1 |
| Eggs | 8.2 |
| Yogurt, plain | 1.5 |
| Ice cream, vanilla | 0.6 |
| Milk, whole | 0.7 |
| | |
| **Fish and Seafood** | |
| Cod | 7.1 |
| Trout | 10.8 |
| | |

| Grain Products | |
| --- | --- |
| Bread, white | 3.7 |
| Bread, whole wheat | 1.8 |
| Rice, brown | 12.5 |
| White flour | 8.2 |
| Spaghetti | 6.5 |

# Chapter 4: Alkaline Diet Recipes

**Breakfast Recipes**

## Raspberry & Banana Smoothie Bowl

**Yield:** 2 servings

**Preparation Time:** 10 minutes

**Total Time:** 10 minutes

**Ingredients:**

- 2 cups fresh raspberries, divided
- 2 large frozen bananas, peeled
- ½ cup unsweetened almond milk
- 1/3 cup fresh mixed berries

**Instructions:**

1. In a blender, add the raspberries, bananas, and almond milk and pulse until smooth.
2. Transfer the smoothie into two serving bowls evenly.
3. Top each bowl with berries and serve immediately.

# Apple & Walnut Porridge

**Yield:** 4 servings

**Preparation Time:** 10 minutes

**Cooking Time:** 5 minutes

**Total Time:** 15 minutes

**Ingredients:**

- 2 cups unsweetened almond milk
- 3 tablespoons walnuts, chopped
- 3 tablespoons sunflower seeds
- 2 large apples, peeled, cored and grated
- ½ teaspoon organic vanilla extract
- Pinch of ground cinnamon
- ½ of small apple, cored and sliced
- 1 small banana, peeled and sliced

**Instructions:**

1. In a large pan, mix together the milk, walnuts, sunflower seeds, grated apple, vanilla and cinnamon over medium-low heat and cook for about 3-5 minutes, stirring frequently.
2. Remove from the heat and transfer the porridge into serving bowls.
3. Top with apple and banana slices and serve.

# Chia Seeds Pudding

**Yield:** 3 servings

**Preparation Time:** 10 minutes

**Total Time:** 10 minutes

**Ingredients:**

- 2 cups unsweetened almond milk
- ½ cup chia seeds
- 1 tablespoon maple syrup
- 1 teaspoon organic vanilla extract
- 1/3 cup fresh strawberries, hulled and sliced
- 2 tablespoons almonds, sliced

**Instructions:**

1. In a large bowl, add the almond milk, chia seeds, maple syrup, and vanilla extract and stir to combine well.
2. Cover the bowl and refrigerate for at least 3-4 hours, stirring occasionally.
3. Serve with the topping of strawberry and almond.

# Cauliflower & Raspberries Porridge

**Yield:** 2 servings

**Preparation Time:** 10 minutes

**Cooking Time:** 15 minutes

**Total Time:** 25 minutes

**Ingredients:**

- 1 cup unsweetened coconut milk
- 1 cup cauliflower rice
- 1/3 cup fresh raspberries
- 3 tablespoons unsweetened coconut, shredded
- 3 drops liquid stevia

**Instructions:**

1. In a pan, add the coconut milk and cauliflower rice over medium heat and cook for about 2-3 minutes, stirring occasionally.
2. Add the raspberries and with the back of a spoon, mash them slightly.
3. Add the coconut and stevia and stir to combine.
4. Cover the pan and cook for about 10 minutes, stirring occasionally.
5. Serve warm.

# Spiced Quinoa Porridge

**Yield:** 4 servings

**Preparation Time:** 10 minutes

**Cooking Time:** 15 minutes

**Total Time:** 25 minutes

**Ingredients:**

- 1 cup uncooked red quinoa, rinsed and drained
- 2 cups alkaline water
- ½ teaspoon organic vanilla extract
- ½ cup coconut milk
- ¼ teaspoon fresh lemon peel, grated finely
- 10-12 drops liquid stevia
- 1 teaspoon ground cinnamon
- ½ teaspoon ground ginger
- Pinch of ground cloves
- 2 tablespoons almonds, chopped

**Instructions:**

1. In a large pan, mix together the quinoa, water, and vanilla extract over medium heat and bring to a boil.
2. Reduce the heat to low and simmer, covered for about 15 minutes or until all the liquid is absorbed, stirring occasionally.

3. In the pan with the quinoa, add the coconut milk, lemon peel, stevia, and spices and stir to combine.

4. Immediately remove from the heat and fluff the quinoa with a fork.

5. Divide the quinoa mixture evenly into serving bowls.

6. Serve with a topping of chopped almonds.

# Chocolaty Quinoa Porridge

**Yield:** 4 servings

**Preparation Time:** 15 minutes

**Cooking Time:** 30 minutes

**Total Time:** 45 minutes

**Ingredients:**

- 1 cup uncooked quinoa, rinsed and drained
- 1 cup unsweetened almond milk
- 1 cup unsweetened coconut milk
- Pinch of sea salt
- 2 tablespoons cacao powder
- 2 tablespoons maple syrup
- ½ teaspoon organic vanilla extract
- ½ cup fresh strawberries, hulled and sliced

**Instructions:**

1. Heat a small non-stick pan over medium heat and cook the quinoa for about 3 minutes or until toasted slightly, stirring frequently.
2. Add the almond milk, coconut milk and a pinch of salt and stir to combine.
3. Increase the heat to high and bring to a boil.

4.  Reduce heat to low and cook, uncovered for about 20-25 minutes or until all the liquid is absorbed, stirring occasionally.

5.  Remove from the heat and immediately, stir in the cacao powder, maple syrup and vanilla extract.

6.  Serve immediately with the topping of strawberry slices.

# Nutty Buckwheat Porridge

**Yield:** 2 servings

**Preparation Time:** 15 minutes

**Cooking Time:** 7 minutes

**Total Time:** 22 minutes

**Ingredients:**

- ½ cup buckwheat groats
- 1 cup alkaline water
- 2 tablespoons chia seeds
- 15-20 almonds
- 1 cup unsweetened almond milk
- ½ teaspoon ground cinnamon
- 1 teaspoon organic vanilla extract
- 3-4 drops liquid stevia
- ¼ cup mixed fresh berries

**Instructions:**

1. In a large bowl, soak buckwheat groats in water overnight.
2. In another 2 bowls, soak chia seeds and almonds respectively.
3. Drain the buckwheat and rinse well.

4. In a non-stick pan, add the buckwheat and almond milk over medium heat and cook for about 7 minutes or until creamy.

5. Drain the chia sees and almonds well.

6. Remove the pan from heat and stir in the almonds, chia seeds, cinnamon, vanilla extract, and stevia.

7. Serve hot with a topping of berries.

# Fruity Oatmeal

**Yield:** 4 servings

**Preparation Time:** 10 minutes

**Cooking Time:** 15 minutes

**Total Time:** 25 minutes

**Ingredients:**

- 4 cups alkaline water
- 1 cup dry steel-cut oats
- 1 large banana, peeled and mashed
- 1½ cups fresh mixed berries (of your choice)
- ¼ cup walnuts, chopped finely

**Instructions:**

1. In a large pan, add the water and oats over medium-high heat and bring to a boil.
2. Reduce the heat to low and simmer for about 20 minutes, stirring occasionally.
3. Remove from heat and cool slightly.
4. Add mashed banana and stir to combine.
5. Top with strawberries and walnuts and serve.

# Baked Nutty Oatmeal

**Yield:** 5 servings

**Preparation Time:** 15 minutes

**Cooking Time:** 45 minutes

**Total Time:** 1 hour

**Ingredients:**

- 1 tablespoon flaxseed meal
- 3 tablespoons alkaline water
- 3 cups unsweetened almond milk
- ¼ cup maple syrup
- 2 tablespoons coconut oil, melted and cooled
- 2 teaspoons organic vanilla extract
- 1 teaspoon ground cinnamon
- 1 teaspoon organic baking powder
- ¼ teaspoon sea salt
- 2 cups old-fashioned rolled oats
- ½ cup almonds, chopped
- ½ cup walnuts, chopped

**Instructions:**

1. Lightly grease an 8x8-inch baking dish. Set aside.
2. In a large bowl, add the flaxseed meal and water and beat until well combined. Set aside for about 5 minutes.

3. In the bowl of flax mixture, add the remaining ingredients except the oats and nuts and mix until well combined.

4. Add the oats and nuts and gently stir to combine.

5. Place the mixture into the prepared baking dish and spread in an even layer.

6. Cover the baking dish with plastic wrap and refrigerate for about 8 hours.

7. Preheat the oven to 350 degrees F. Arrange a rack in the middle of the oven.

8. Remove the baking dish from the refrigerator and let sit at room temperature for 15-20 minutes.

9. Remove the plastic wrap and stir the oatmeal mixture well.

10. Bake for about 45 minutes.

11. Remove from the oven and set aside to cool slightly.

12. Serve warm.

# Banana Waffles

**Yield:** 5 servings

**Preparation Time:** 15 minutes

**Cooking Time:** 20 minutes

**Total Time:** 35 minutes

**Ingredients:**

- 2 tablespoons flax meal
- 6 tablespoons warm alkaline water
- 2 bananas, peeled and mashed
- 1 cup creamy almond butter
- ¼ cup full-fat coconut milk

**Instructions:**

1. In a small bowl, add the flax meal and warm water and beat until well combined.
2. Set aside for about 10 minutes or until mixture becomes thick.
3. In a medium mixing bowl, add the bananas, almond butter, and coconut milk, mix well.
4. Add the flax meal mixture and mix until well combined.
5. Preheat the waffle iron and lightly grease it.
6. Place desired amount of the mixture in the preheated waffle iron.

7.  Cook for about 3-4 minutes or until waffles become golden brown.

8.  Repeat with the remaining mixture.

9.  Serve warm.

# Savory Sweet Potato Waffles

**Yield:** 2 servings

**Preparation Time:** 10 minutes

**Cooking Time:** 20 minutes

**Total Time:** 30 minutes

**Ingredients:**

- 1 medium sweet potato, peeled, grated and squeezed
- 1 teaspoon fresh thyme, minced
- 1 teaspoon fresh rosemary, minced
- 1/8 teaspoon red pepper flakes, crushed
- Sea salt and freshly ground black pepper, to taste

**Instructions:**

1. Preheat the waffle iron and then grease it.
2. In a large bowl, add all the ingredients and mix until well combined.
3. Place ½ of the sweet potato mixture into the preheated waffle iron and cook for about 8-10 minutes or until golden brown.
4. Repeat with the remaining mixture.
5. Serve warm.

# Fruity Oat Pancakes

**Yield:** 3 servings

**Preparation Time:** 10 minutes

**Cooking Time:** 15 minutes

**Total Time:** 25 minutes

**Ingredients:**

- 1 cup rolled oats
- 1 medium banana, peeled and mashed
- ¼-½ cup unsweetened almond milk
- 1 tablespoon organic baking powder
- 1 tablespoon organic apple cider vinegar
- 1 tablespoon agave nectar
- ½ teaspoon organic vanilla extract
- ½ cup fresh blackberries

**Instructions:**

1. Place all the ingredients except the blackberries in a large bowl and mix until well combined.
2. Gently fold in the blackberries.
3. Set the mixture aside for about 5-10 minutes.
4. Preheat a large non-stick skillet over medium-low heat.
5. Add about ¼ cup of the mixture and with a spatula, spread in an even layer.

6. Immediately, cover the skillet and cook for about 2-3 minutes or until golden brown.

7. Flip the pancake over and cook for 1-2 minutes more or until golden brown.

8. Repeat with the remaining mixture.

9. Serve warm.

# Tofu & Mushroom Muffins

**Yield:** 6 servings

**Preparation Time:** 15 minutes

**Cooking Time:** 30 minutes

**Total Time:** 45 minutes

**Ingredients:**

- 1 teaspoon olive oil
- 1½ cups fresh button mushrooms, chopped
- 1 scallion, chopped
- 1 teaspoon garlic, minced
- 1 teaspoon fresh rosemary, minced
- Freshly ground black pepper, to taste
- 1 (12.3-ounce) package firm silken tofu, drained, pressed and sliced
- ¼ cup unsweetened almond milk
- 2 tablespoons nutritional yeast
- 1 tablespoon arrowroot starch
- ¼ teaspoon ground turmeric
- 1 teaspoon coconut oil, softened

**Instructions:**

1. Preheat the oven to 375 degrees F. Grease a 12-cup muffin pan.

2. In a non-stick skillet, heat oil over medium heat and sauté scallion and garlic for about 1 minute.

3. Add the mushrooms and cook for about 5-7 minutes, stirring frequently.

4. Stir in the rosemary and black pepper and remove from the heat.

5. Set aside to cool slightly.

6. In a food processor, add the tofu and remaining ingredients and pulse until smooth.

7. Transfer the tofu mixture into a large bowl.

8. Fold in the mushroom mixture.

9. Divide the tofu mixture into the prepared muffin cups evenly.

10. Bake for 20-22 minutes or until a toothpick inserted in the center comes out clean.

11. Remove the muffin pan from oven and place onto a wire rack to cool for about 10 minutes.

12. Carefully invert the muffins onto the wire rack and serve warm.

# Simple White Bread

**Yield:** 8 servings

**Preparation Time:** 10 minutes

**Cooking Time:** 1 hour 10 minutes

**Total Time:** 1 hour 20 minutes

**Ingredients:**

- 4 cups spelt flour
- 4 tablespoons sesame seeds
- 1 teaspoon baking soda
- ¼ teaspoon sea salt
- 10-12 drops liquid stevia
- 2 cups plus 2 tablespoons unsweetened almond milk

**Instructions:**

1. Preheat the oven to 350 degrees F. Line a 9x5-inch loaf pan with a greased parchment paper.
2. In a large bowl, add all the ingredients and with a fork, mix until well combined.
3. Transfer the mixture in prepared loaf pan evenly.
4. Bake for about 70 minutes or until a toothpick inserted in the center comes out clean.
5. Remove from oven and place the loaf pan onto a wire rack to cool for at least 10 minutes.

6. Carefully, invert the bread loaf onto the wire rack to cool completely before slicing.

7. With a sharp knife, cut the bread loaf into desired sized slices and serve.

# Quinoa Bread

**Yield:** 12 servings

**Preparation Time:** 10 minutes

**Cooking Time:** 1½ hours

**Total Time:** 1 hour 40 minutes

**Ingredients:**

- ¼ cup chia seeds
- 1 cup alkaline water, divided
- 1¾ cups uncooked quinoa, soaked overnight and rinsed
- ½ teaspoon bicarbonate soda
- ¼ teaspoon sea salt
- ¼ cup olive oil
- 1 tablespoon fresh lemon juice

**Instructions:**

1. In a bowl, soak chia seeds in ½ cup of water overnight,
2. Preheat the oven to 320 degrees F. Line a loaf pan with parchment paper.
3. In a food processor, add the chia seed mixture and remaining ingredients and pulse for about 3 minutes.
4. Place the bread mixture into the prepared loaf pan evenly.
5. Bake for about 1½ hours or until a toothpick inserted in the center comes out clean.

6. Remove the bread pan from oven and place onto a wire rack to cool for about 10 minutes.

7. Carefully, invert the bread loaf onto the wire rack to cool completely before slicing.

8. With a sharp knife, cut the bread loaf into desired sized slices and serve.

# Zucchini & Banana Bread

**Yield:** 6 servings

**Preparation Time:** 15 minutes

**Cooking Time:** 45 minutes

**Total Time:** 1 hour

**Ingredients:**

- ½ cup almond flour, sifted
- 1½ teaspoons baking soda
- ½ teaspoon ground cinnamon
- ¼ teaspoon ground cardamom
- 1/8 teaspoon ground cloves
- 1½ cups banana, peeled and sliced
- ¼ cup almond butter, softened
- 2 teaspoons organic vanilla extract
- 1 cup zucchini, shredded and squeezed

**Instructions:**

1. Preheat oven to 350 degrees F. Grease a 6x3-inch loaf pan.
2. In a large bowl, add the flour, baking soda and spices and with a fork, mix well.
3. In another bowl, add the banana and with a fork, mash it completely.

4.  In the bowl of banana, add the almond butter and vanilla extract and beat until well combined.

5.  Add the flour mixture and mix until just combined.

6.  Gently, fold in the grated zucchini.

7.  Place the flour mixture into the prepared loaf pan evenly.

8.  Bake for about 40-45 minutes or until a toothpick inserted in the center comes out clean.

9.  Remove from oven and place the loaf pan onto a wire rack to cool for at least 10 minutes.

10. Carefully, invert the bread onto the rack to cool completely before slicing.

11. With a sharp knife, cut the bread loaf into desired sized slices and serve.

# Tofu & Veggie Scramble

**Yield:** 2 servings

**Preparation Time:** 15 minutes

**Cooking Time:** 15 minutes

**Total Time:** 30 minutes

**Ingredients:**

- ½ tablespoon olive oil
- 1 small onion, chopped finely
- 1 small red bell pepper, seeded and chopped finely
- 1 cup cherry tomatoes, chopped finely
- 1½ cups firm tofu, drained, pressed and chopped
- Pinch of cayenne pepper
- Pinch of ground turmeric
- Sea salt, to taste
- 1 tablespoon fresh basil, chopped

**Instructions:**

1. In a skillet, heat oil over medium heat and sauté the onion and bell pepper for about 4-5 minutes.
2. Add the tomatoes and cook for about 1-2 minutes, stirring occasionally.
3. Add the tofu, turmeric, cayenne pepper and salt and cook for about 6-8 minutes, stirring frequently. '
4. Serve hot with the garnishing of basil.

# Eggless Tomato Omelet

**Yield:** 4 servings

**Preparation Time:** 15 minutes

**Cooking Time:** 25 minutes

**Total Time:** 40 minutes

**Ingredients:**

- 1 cup chickpea flour
- ¼ teaspoon ground turmeric
- ¼ teaspoon red chili powder
- Pinch of ground cumin
- Sea salt and freshly ground black pepper, to taste
- 1½-2 cups alkaline water
- 1 medium white onion, chopped finely
- 2 medium fresh tomatoes, chopped finely
- 1 small jalapeño pepper, seeded and chopped finely
- 2 tablespoons fresh parsley, chopped
- 2 tablespoons olive oil, divided

**Instructions:**

1. In a large bowl, add the flour, spices, salt and black pepper and with a fork, mix well.
2. Slowly add the water and mix until well combined.

3.  Add the onion, tomatoes, green chili, and parsley and gently stir to combine.
4.  In a large non-stick frying pan, heat ½ tablespoon of oil over medium heat.
5.  Add ½ of tomato mixture and tilt the pan to spread in an even layer.
6.  Cook for about 5-7 minutes.
7.  Pour the remaining oil on top and carefully flip the omelet.
8.  Cook for about 4-5 minutes or until golden brown and remove from pan.
9.  Carefully, transfer the omelet onto a serving plate.
10. Repeat with the remaining mixture.
11. Serve warm.

# Eggless Veggies Omelet

**Yield:** 2 servings

**Preparation Time:** 20 minutes

**Cooking Time:** 23 minutes

**Total Time:** 43 minutes

**Ingredients:**

- 8 ounces fresh asparagus, trimmed and cut into 1-inch slices
- ¼ of red bell pepper, seeded and chopped
- ¼ of green bell pepper, seeded and chopped
- 1 tablespoon fresh chives, chopped
- ¾ cup alkaline water
- ½ cup superfine chickpea flour
- 1 tablespoon chia seeds
- 2 tablespoons nutritional yeast
- ½ teaspoon organic baking powder
- 1 teaspoon dried basil, crushed
- ¼ teaspoon ground turmeric
- ¼ teaspoon red pepper flakes, crushed
- Sea salt and freshly ground black pepper, to taste
- 1 small tomato, chopped

**Instructions:**

1. In a pan of lightly salted boiling water, add the asparagus and cook for about 5-7 minutes or until crisp tender.
2. Drain the asparagus well and set aside.
3. Meanwhile, in a bowl, add the bell peppers, chives and water and mix well.
4. In another bowl, add the remaining ingredients except tomato and mix well.
5. Add the bell pepper mixture into flour mixture and mix until well combined.
6. Set aside for at least 10 minutes.
7. Lightly, grease a charge non-stick skillet and heat over medium heat.
8. Add ½ of the mixture and with a back of a spoon, smooth it.
9. Sprinkle half of tomato over mixture evenly.
10. With the lid, cover the skillet tightly and cook for about 4 minutes.
11. Uncover the skillet and place half of cooked asparagus over one side of omelet.
12. Carefully, fold the other half over asparagus to cover it.
13. Cover the skillet and cook for about 3-4 minutes more.
14. Repeat with the remaining mixture.
15. Serve warm.

# Coconut, Nuts & Seeds Granola

**Yield:** 8 servings

**Preparation Time:** 15 minutes

**Cooking Time:** 23 minutes

**Total Time:** 43 minutes

**Ingredients:**

- ½ cup unsweetened coconut flakes
- 1 cup raw almonds
- 1 cup raw walnuts
- ½ cup raw sunflower seeds, shelled
- ¼ cup coconut oil
- ½ cup maple syrup
- 1 teaspoon organic vanilla extract
- ½ cup golden raisins
- ½ cup black raisins
- Sea salt, to taste

**Instructions:**

1. Preheat the oven to 275 F. Line a large baking sheet with parchment paper.
2. In a food processor, add the coconut flakes, almonds, walnuts, and seeds and pulse until chopped finely.

3.  Meanwhile, in a medium non-stick pan, add the oil, maple syrup, and vanilla extract and cook for 3 minutes over medium-high heat stirring continuously.
4.  Remove from the heat and immediately stir in the nut mixture.
5.  Transfer the mixture to the prepared baking sheet and spread it out evenly.
6.  Bake for about 25 minutes, stirring twice.
7.  Remove the pan from the oven and immediately stir in the raisins.
8.  Sprinkle with a little salt.
9.  With the back of a spatula, flatten the surface of the mixture.
10. Set aside to cool completely.
11. Then, break the granola into even-sized chunks.
12. Serve this granola with your choice of non-dairy milk and fruit topping.
13. For preserving, transfer this granola to an airtight container and keep it in the refrigerator.

# Smoothie Recipes

## Banana & Almond Smoothie

**Yield:** 2 servings

**Preparation Time:** 10 minutes

**Total Time:** 10 minutes

**Ingredients:**

- 2 large frozen bananas, peeled and sliced
- 1 tablespoon almonds, chopped
- 1 teaspoon organic vanilla extract
- 2 cups chilled unsweetened almond milk

**Instructions:**

1. Place all the ingredients in a high-speed blender and pulse until smooth and creamy.
2. Pour the smoothie into two serving glasses and serve immediately.

# Strawberry & Beet Smoothie

**Yield:** 2 servings

**Preparation Time:** 10 minutes

**Total Time:** 10 minutes

**Ingredients:**

- 2 cups frozen strawberries, hulled
- 2/3 cup frozen beets, trimmed, peeled and chopped
- 1 teaspoon fresh ginger root, peeled and grated
- 1 teaspoon fresh turmeric root, peeled and grated
- ½ cup fresh orange juice
- 1 cup unsweetened almond milk

**Instructions:**

1. Place all the ingredients in a high-speed blender and pulse until smooth and creamy.
2. Pour the smoothie into two serving glasses and serve immediately.

# Raspberry & Tofu Smoothie

**Yield:** 2 servings

**Preparation Time:** 10 minutes

**Total Time:** 10 minutes

**Ingredients:**

- 1½ cups fresh raspberries
- 6 ounces firm silken tofu, drained, pressed and chopped
- 1 teaspoon powdered stevia
- 1/8 teaspoon organic vanilla extract
- 1½ cups unsweetened almond milk
- ¼ cup ice cubes, crushed

**Instructions:**

1. Place all the ingredients in a high-speed blender and pulse until smooth and creamy.
2. Pour the smoothie into two serving glasses and serve immediately.

# Lemony Mango Smoothie

**Yield:** 2 servings

**Preparation Time:** 10 minutes

**Total Time:** 10 minutes

**Ingredients:**

- 2 cups frozen mango, peeled, pitted and chopped
- ¼ cup almond butter
- Pinch of ground turmeric
- 2 tablespoons fresh lemon juice
- 1¼ cups unsweetened almond milk
- ¼ cup ice cubes, crushed

**Instructions:**

1. Place all the ingredients in a high-speed blender and pulse until smooth and creamy.
2. Pour the smoothie into two serving glasses and serve immediately.

# Papaya & Banana Smoothie

**Yield:** 2 servings

**Preparation Time:** 10 minutes

**Total Time:** 10 minutes

**Ingredients:**

- ½ of medium papaya, peeled and chopped roughly
- 1 large banana, peeled and sliced
- 2 tablespoons agave nectar
- ¼ teaspoon ground turmeric
- 1 tablespoon fresh lime juice
- 1½ cups unsweetened almond milk
- ½ cup ice cubes, crushed

**Instructions:**

1. Place all the ingredients in a high-speed blender and pulse until smooth and creamy.
2. Pour the smoothie into two serving glasses and serve immediately.

# Orange & Oats Smoothie

**Yield:** 2 servings

**Preparation Time:** 10 minutes

**Total Time:** 10 minutes

**Ingredients:**

- 2/3 cups rolled oats
- 2 oranges, peeled, seeded, and sectioned
- 2 large bananas, peeled and sliced
- 1½ cups unsweetened almond milk
- ½ cup ice cubes, crushed

**Instructions:**

1. Place all the ingredients in a high-speed blender and pulse until smooth and creamy.
2. Pour the smoothie into two serving glasses and serve immediately.

# Pineapple & Kale Smoothie

**Yield:** 2 servings

**Preparation Time:** 10 minutes

**Total Time:** 10 minutes

**Ingredients:**

- 1½ cups fresh kale, tough ribs removed and chopped
- 1 large frozen banana, peeled and sliced
- ½ cup fresh pineapple, peeled and cut into chunks
- ½ cup fresh orange juice
- 1 cup unsweetened coconut milk
- ½ cup ice cubes, crushed

**Instructions:**

1. Place all the ingredients in a high-speed blender and pulse until smooth and creamy.
2. Pour the smoothie into two serving glasses and serve immediately.

# Pumpkin & Banana Smoothie

**Yield:** 2 servings

**Preparation Time:** 10 minutes

**Total Time:** 10 minutes

**Ingredients:**

- 1 cup homemade pumpkin puree
- 1 large banana, peeled and sliced
- 1 tablespoon maple syrup
- 1 teaspoon ground flaxseeds
- ¼ teaspoon ground cinnamon
- 1/8 teaspoon ground ginger
- 1½ cups unsweetened almond milk
- ¼ cup ice cubes, crushed

**Instructions:**

1. Place all the ingredients in a high-speed blender and pulse until smooth and creamy.
2. Pour the smoothie into two serving glasses and serve immediately.

# Kale & Avocado Smoothie

**Yield:** 2 servings

**Preparation Time:** 10 minutes

**Total Time:** 10 minutes

**Ingredients:**

- 2 cups fresh kale, tough ribs removed and chopped
- ½ of medium avocado, peeled, pitted and chopped
- ½-inch pieces fresh ginger root, peeled and chopped
- ½-inch pieces fresh turmeric root, peeled and chopped
- 1½ cups unsweetened coconut milk
- ¼ cup ice cubes, crushed

**Instructions:**

1. Place all the ingredients in a high-speed blender and pulse until smooth and creamy.
2. Pour the smoothie into two serving glasses and serve immediately.

# Herbed Cucumber & Greens Smoothie

**Yield:** 2 servings

**Preparation Time:** 10 minutes

**Total Time:** 10 minutes

**Ingredients:**

- 2 cups mixed fresh greens (kale, beet greens), trimmed and chopped
- 1 small cucumber, peeled and chopped
- ½ cup lettuce, torn
- ¼ cup fresh parsley leaves
- ¼ cup fresh mint leaves
- 2-3 drops liquid stevia
- 1 teaspoon fresh lemon juice
- 1½ cups alkaline water
- ¼ cup ice cubes, crushed

**Instructions:**

1. Place all the ingredients in a high-speed blender and pulse until smooth and creamy.
2. Pour the smoothie into two serving glasses and serve immediately.

# Green Veggies & Avocado Smoothie

**Yield:** 2 servings

**Preparation Time:** 15 minutes

**Total Time:** 15 minutes

**Ingredients:**

- 1 medium avocado, peeled, pitted and chopped
- 1 large cucumber, peeled and chopped
- 2 fresh tomatoes, chopped
- 1 small green bell pepper, seeded and chopped
- 1 cup fresh kale, tough ribs removed and torn
- 2 tablespoons fresh lime juice
- 2 tablespoons homemade vegetable broth
- 1 cup alkaline water
- ¼ cup ice cubes, crushed

**Instructions:**

1. Place all the ingredients in a high-speed blender and pulse until smooth and creamy.
2. Pour the smoothie into two serving glasses and serve immediately.

# Green Tofu & Veggie Smoothie

**Yield:** 2 servings

**Preparation Time:** 10 minutes

**Total Time:** 10 minutes

**Ingredients:**

- 1½ cups cucumber, peeled and chopped roughly
- 3 cups fresh baby kale
- 1 cup frozen broccoli
- ½ cup silken tofu, drained, pressed and chopped
- 1 tablespoon fresh lime juice
- 4-5 drops liquid stevia
- 1 cup unsweetened almond milk
- ½ cup ice cubes, crushed

**Instructions:**

1. Place all the ingredients in a high-speed blender and pulse until smooth and creamy.
2. Pour the smoothie into two serving glasses and serve immediately.

# Red Fruit & Veggies Smoothie

**Yield:** 2 servings

**Preparation Time:** 10 minutes

**Total Time:** 10 minutes

**Ingredients:**

- ½ cup fresh raspberries
- ½ cup fresh strawberries, hulled
- ½ of red bell pepper, seeded and chopped
- ½ cup red cabbage, chopped
- 1 small tomato, chopped
- 1¼ cups alkaline water
- ½ cup ice cubes

**Instructions:**

1. Place all the ingredients in a high-speed blender and pulse until smooth and creamy.
2. Pour the smoothie into two serving glasses and serve immediately.

# Lunch Recipes

## Veggie Lettuce Wraps

**Yield:** 4 servings

**Preparation Time:** 20 minutes

**Cooking Time:** 10 minutes

**Total Time:** 30 minutes

**Ingredients:**

**For Filling:**

- 1 teaspoon olive oil
- 2 cups fresh shiitake mushrooms, chopped
- 2 teaspoons tamari, divided
- 1 cup cooked quinoa
- 1 teaspoon fresh lime juice
- 1 teaspoon organic apple cider vinegar
- ¼ cup scallion, chopped
- Sea salt and freshly ground black pepper, to taste

**For Creamy Sauce:**

- 5 ounces silken tofu, pressed, drained and chopped
- 1 small garlic clove, chopped
- ¼ cup smooth almond butter
- 1 teaspoon fresh lime juice

- Sea salt and freshly ground black pepper, to taste

## For Wraps:

- 8 medium butter lettuce leaves
- ¼ cup cucumber, peeled and julienned
- ¼ cup carrot, peeled and julienned
- ¼ cup cabbage, shredded

## Instructions:

1. For filling in a skillet, heat the oil over medium heat and cook the mushrooms and 1 teaspoon of tamari for about 5-8 minutes, stirring frequently.
2. Stir in the quinoa, lime juice, vinegar and remaining tamari and cook for about 1 minute, stirring continuously.
3. Stir in the scallion, salt and black pepper and immediately, remove from heat.
4. Set aside to cool.
5. Meanwhile, for sauce: in a food processor, add all ingredients and pulse until smooth.
6. Arrange the lettuce leaves onto serving plates.
7. Place quinoa filling over each leaf evenly and top with cucumber, carrot and cabbage.
8. Serve alongside the creamy sauce.

# Oat, Tofu & Spinach Burgers

**Yield:** 4 servings

**Preparation Time:** 15 minutes

**Cooking Time:** 16 minutes

**Total Time:** 31 minutes

**Ingredients:**

- 1 pound firm tofu, drained, pressed, and crumbled
- ¾ cup rolled oats
- ¼ cup flaxseeds
- 2 cups frozen kale, thawed, squeezed and chopped
- 1 medium onion, chopped finely
- 4 garlic cloves, minced
- 1 teaspoon ground cumin
- 1 teaspoon red pepper flakes, crushed
- Sea salt and freshly ground black pepper, to taste
- 2 tablespoons olive oil
- 6 cups fresh salad greens

**Instructions:**

1. In a large bowl, add all the ingredients except oil and salad greens and mix until well combined.
2. Set aside for about 10 minutes.
3. Make desired sized patties from the mixture.

4.  In a non-stick frying pan, heat the oil over medium heat
    and cook the patties for 6-8 minutes per side.
5.  Serve these patties alongside the salad greens.

# Beans, Walnuts & Veggies Burgers

**Yield:** 4 servings

**Preparation Time:** 20 minutes

**Cooking Time:** 25 minutes

**Total Time:** 45 minutes

**Ingredients:**

- ½ cup walnuts
- 1 carrot, peeled and chopped
- 1 celery stalk, chopped
- 4 scallions, chopped
- 5 garlic cloves, chopped
- 2¼ cups canned black beans, rinsed and drained
- 2½ cups sweet potato, peeled and grated
- ½ teaspoon red pepper flakes, crushed
- ¼ teaspoon cayenne pepper
- Sea salt and freshly ground black pepper, to taste
- 12 cups fresh baby greens

**Instructions:**

1. Preheat the oven to 400 degrees F. Line a baking sheet with parchment paper.
2. In a food processor, add the walnuts and pulse until finely ground.

3. Add the carrot, celery, scallion and garlic and pulse until chopped finely.

4. Transfer the vegetable mixture into a large bowl.

5. In the same food processor, add the beans and pulse until chopped.

6. Add 1½ cups of the sweet potato and pulse until a chunky mixture forms.

7. Transfer the bean mixture into the bowl with vegetable mixture.

8. Stir in the remaining sweet potato, spices, salt and black pepper and mix until well combined.

9. Make 8 equal-sized patties from the beans mixture.

10. Arrange the patties onto the prepared baking sheet in a single layer.

11. Bake for about 25 minutes.

12. Divide the greens onto serving plates and top each with 2 patties.

13. Serve immediately.

# Tofu & Broccoli Stuffed Avocados

**Yield:** 6 servings

**Preparation Time:** 20 minutes

**Cooking Time:** 15 minutes

**Total Time:** 35 minutes

**Ingredients:**

**For Marinade:**

- ¼ cup fresh parsley leaves, chopped
- 1 small garlic clove, minced
- 1 teaspoon fresh lemon zest, grated finely
- 1 tablespoon Dijon mustard
- ¼ cup olive oil
- 2 tablespoons fresh lemon juice
- ¼ teaspoon ground cumin
- Sea salt and freshly ground black pepper, to taste
- 1 (8-ounce) package firm tofu, drained, pressed and cut into ½-inch slices
- 1 cup small broccoli florets

**For Stuffed Avocados:**

- 1 tablespoon fresh chives, minced
- 3 firm avocados, peeled, halved and pitted
- Sea salt and freshly ground black pepper, to taste

- 2 tablespoons fresh parsley, chopped

**Instructions:**

1. For marinade: in a large bowl, add all the ingredients except tofu and beat until well combined.
2. Add the tofu and broccoli and coat with the marinade generously.
3. Cover the bowl and refrigerate for about 1 hour.
4. Preheat the grill to medium-high heat. Generously, grease the grill grate.
5. Place the tofu slices onto the grill and cook for about 2 minutes per side.
6. Grill the broccoli florets for about 8-10 minutes, flipping occasionally.
7. Remove the tofu and broccoli from the grill and transfer into a large bowl.
8. Set aside to cool slightly.
9. Then, chop the tofu and broccoli into tiny pieces.
10. Transfer the tofu and broccoli into a bowl with the chives and mix well.
11. Sprinkle the avocado halves with salt and black pepper.
12. Stuff each half with tofu mixture evenly.
13. Garnish with parsley and serve immediately.

# Nutty Brussels Sprout

**Yield:** 2 servings

**Preparation Time:** 15 minutes

**Cooking Time:** 15 minutes

**Total Time:** 30 minutes

**Ingredients:**

- ½ pound Brussels sprouts, trimmed and halved
- 1 tablespoon olive oil
- 2 garlic cloves, minced
- ½ teaspoon red pepper flakes, crushed
- Sea salt and freshly ground black pepper, to taste
- 1 tablespoon fresh lemon juice
- 1 tablespoon pine nuts

**Instructions:**

1. In a large pan of the boiling water, arrange a steamer basket.
2. Place the asparagus in steamer basket and steam, covered for about 6-8 minutes.
3. Drain the asparagus well.
4. In a large skillet, heat the oil over medium heat and sauté the garlic and red pepper flakes for about 30-40 seconds.
5. Stir in the Brussels sprouts, salt and black pepper and sauté for about 4-5 minutes.

6.  Stir in the lemon juice and sauté for about 1 minute more.

7.  Stir in the pine nuts and remove from the heat.

8.  Serve hot.

# Broccoli with Kale

**Yield:** 8 servings

**Preparation Time:** 20 minutes

**Cooking Time:** 1 hour 20 minutes

**Total Time:** 1 hour 40 minutes

**Ingredients:**

- 3 tablespoons coconut oil, divided
- ¼ of small yellow onion, chopped
- 1 teaspoon garlic, minced
- 1 teaspoon fresh ginger root, peeled and minced
- 1 cup broccoli florets
- 2 cups fresh kale, tough ribs removed and chopped
- ½ cup coconut cream
- ¼ teaspoon red pepper flakes, crushed
- 1 teaspoon fresh parsley, chopped finely

**Instructions:**

1. In a large skillet, melt 2 tablespoons of the coconut oil over medium-high heat and sauté the onion for about 3-4 minutes.
2. Add the garlic and ginger and sauté for about 1 minute.
3. Add the broccoli and stir to combine well.
4. Immediately, reduce the heat to medium-low and cook for about 2-3 minutes, stirring continuously.

5. Stir in the kale and cook or about 3 minutes, stirring frequently.

6. Add the coconut cream and remaining coconut oil and stir until smooth.

7. Stir in the red pepper flakes and simmer for about 5-10 minutes, stirring occasionally or until the desired thickness of the curry.

8. Remove from the heat and serve hot with the topping of parsley.

# Parsley Mushrooms

**Yield:** 2 servings

**Preparation Time:** 15 minutes

**Cooking Time:** 15 minutes

**Total Time:** 30 minutes

**Ingredients:**

- 2 tablespoons olive oil
- 2-3 tablespoons onion, minced
- ½ teaspoon garlic, minced
- 12 ounces fresh mushrooms, sliced
- 1 tablespoon fresh parsley, chopped
- Sea salt and freshly ground black pepper, to taste

**Instructions:**

1. In a skillet, heat the oil over medium heat and sauté the onion and garlic for 2-3 minutes.
2. Add the mushrooms and cook for 8-10 minutes or until desired doneness, stirring frequently.
3. Stir in the parsley salt and black pepper and remove from the heat.
4. Serve hot.

# Garlicky Broccoli

**Yield:** 3 servings

**Preparation Time:** 15 minutes

**Cooking Time:** 8 minutes

**Total Time:** 23 minutes

**Ingredients:**

- 1 tablespoon olive oil
- 2 garlic cloves, minced
- 2 cups broccoli florets
- 2 tablespoons alkaline water
- Sea salt and freshly ground black pepper, to taste

**Instructions:**

1. In a large skillet, heat the oil over medium heat and sauté the garlic for about 1 minute.
2. Add the broccoli and stir fry for about 2 minutes.
3. Stir in the water, salt and black pepper and stir fry for 4-5 minutes.
4. Remove from the heat and serve hot.

# Broccoli with Bell Pepper

**Yield:** 5 servings

**Preparation Time:** 15 minutes

**Cooking Time:** 10 minutes

**Total Time:** 25 minutes

**Ingredients:**

- 2 tablespoons olive oil
- 4 garlic cloves, minced
- 1 large white onion, sliced
- 2 cups small broccoli florets
- 3 red bell peppers, seeded and sliced
- ¼ cup homemade vegetable broth
- Sea salt and freshly ground black pepper, to taste

**Instructions:**

1. In a large skillet, heat the oil over medium heat and sauté the garlic for about 1 minute.
2. Add the onion, broccoli and bell peppers and stir fry for about 5 minutes.
3. Add the broth and stir fry for about 4 minutes more.
4. Serve hot.

# Spiced Okra

**Yield:** 2 servings

**Preparation Time:** 15 minutes

**Cooking Time:** 13 minutes

**Total Time:** 28 minutes

**Ingredients:**

- 1 tablespoon olive oil
- ½ teaspoon cumin seeds
- ¾ pound okra pods, trimmed and cut into 2-inch pieces
- ½ teaspoon red chili powder
- 1 teaspoon ground coriander
- Sea salt and freshly ground black pepper, to taste

**Instructions:**

1. In a large skillet, heat the oil over medium heat and sauté the cumin seeds for 30 seconds.
2. Add the okra and stir fry for 1-1½ minutes.
3. Reduce the heat to low and cook, covered for 6-8 minutes, stirring occasionally.
4. Uncover and increase the heat to medium.
5. Stir in the chili powder and coriander and cook for 2-3 more minutes.
6. Season with the salt and remove from heat.
7. Serve hot.

## Spicy Cauliflower

**Yield:** 4 servings

**Preparation Time:** 15 minutes

**Cooking Time:** 20 minutes

**Total Time:** 35 minutes

**Ingredients:**

- ¼ cup alkaline water
- 2 medium fresh tomatoes, chopped
- 2 tablespoons extra-virgin olive oil
- 1 small white onion, chopped
- ½ tablespoon fresh ginger root, peeled and minced
- 3 medium garlic cloves, minced
- 1 jalapeño pepper, seeded and chopped
- 1 teaspoon ground cumin
- 1 teaspoon ground coriander
- 1 teaspoon cayenne pepper
- ¼ teaspoon ground turmeric
- 3 cups cauliflower, chopped
- Sea salt and freshly ground black pepper, to taste
- ½ cup warm alkaline water
- ¼ cup fresh parsley leaves, chopped

## Instructions:

1. In a blender, add ¼ cup of water and tomatoes and pulse until pureed. Set aside.
2. In a large skillet, heat the oil over medium heat and sauté the onion for about 4-5 minutes.
3. Add the ginger, garlic, jalapeño pepper and spices and sauté for about 1 minute.
4. Add the tomato puree and cauliflower and cook for about 3-4 minutes, stirring continuously.
5. Add the warm water and bring to a boil.
6. Reduce the heat to medium-low and simmer, covered for about 8-10 minutes or until desired doneness of cauliflower.
7. Remove from the heat and serve hot with the garnishing of parsley.

# Eggplant Curry

**Yield:** 3 servings

**Preparation Time:** 15 minutes

**Cooking Time:** 35 minutes

**Total Time:** 50 minutes

**Ingredients:**

- 1 tablespoon coconut oil
- 1 medium onion, chopped finely
- 2 garlic cloves, minced
- ½ tablespoon fresh ginger root, peeled and minced
- 1 Serrano pepper, seeded and minced
- Sea salt and freshly ground black pepper, to taste
- 1 medium tomato, chopped finely
- 1 large eggplant, cubed
- 1 cup unsweetened coconut milk
- 2 tablespoons fresh parsley, chopped

**Instructions:**

1. In a large skillet, melt the coconut oil over medium heat and sauté the onion for 8-9 minutes.
2. Add the garlic, garlic, Serrano pepper and salt and sauté for 1 minute.
3. Add the tomato and cook for 3-4 minutes, crushing with the back of a spoon.

4. Add the eggplant and salt and cook for 1 minute, stirring occasionally.

5. Stir in the coconut milk and bring to a gentle boil.

6. Reduce the heat to medium-low and simmer, covered for 15-20 minutes or until done completely.

7. Remove from the heat and serve with the garnishing of parsley.

# Lemony Kale with Scallions

**Yield:** 4 servings

**Preparation Time:** 15 minutes

**Cooking Time:** 20 minutes

**Total Time:** 35 minutes

**Ingredients:**

- 1 tablespoon extra-virgin olive oil
- 1 lemon, seeded and sliced thinly
- 1 white onion, sliced thinly
- 3 garlic cloves, minced
- 2 pounds fresh kale, tough ribs removed and chopped
- ½ cup scallions, chopped
- Sea salt and freshly ground black pepper, to taste

**Instructions:**

1. In a large skillet, heat the oil over medium heat and cook the lemon slices for 5 minutes.
2. With a slotted spoon, remove the lemon slices from skillet and set aside.
3. In the same skillet, add the onion and garlic and sauté for about 5 minutes.
4. Add the kale, scallions, salt, and pepper and cook for 8-10 minutes.
5. Add the lemon slices and mix until well combined.

6.  Remove from the heat and serve hot.

# Veggies with Apple

**Yield:** 4 servings

**Preparation Time:** 15 minutes

**Cooking Time:** 16 minutes

**Total Time:** 31 minutes

**Ingredients:**

**For Sauce:**

- 3 small garlic cloves, minced
- 1 teaspoon fresh ginger root, peeled and minced
- 1 tablespoon fresh orange zest, grated finely
- ½ cup fresh orange juice
- 1 tablespoon maple syrup
- 2 tablespoons tamari
- 2 tablespoons organic apple cider vinegar

**For Veggies & Apple:**

- 1 tablespoon olive oil
- 2 cups carrot, peeled and julienned
- 1 head broccoli, cut into florets
- 1 cup red onion, chopped
- 2 apples, cored and sliced

**Instructions:**

1. For sauce: in a large bowl, add all the ingredients and with a wire whisk, beat until well combined. Set aside.
2. In a large skillet, heat the oil over medium-high heat and stir fry the carrot and broccoli for about 4-5 minutes.
3. Add the onion and stir fry for about 4-5 minutes.
4. Stir in sauce and cook for about 2-3 minutes, stirring frequently.
5. Stir in the apple slices and cook for about 2-3 minutes.
6. Remove from the heat and serve hot.

# Cabbage with Apple

**Yield:** 4 servings

**Preparation Time:** 15 minutes

**Cooking Time:** 12 minutes

**Total Time:** 27 minutes

**Ingredients:**

- 2 teaspoons coconut oil
- 1 large apple, cored and sliced thinly
- 1 onion, sliced thinly
- 1½ pounds cabbage, chopped finely
- 1 tablespoon fresh thyme, chopped
- 1 fresh red chili, chopped
- 1 tablespoon organic apple cider vinegar

**Instructions:**

1. In a non-stick skillet, melt 1 teaspoon of coconut oil over medium heat and stir fry apple for about 2-3 minutes.
2. Transfer the apple into a bowl.
3. In the same skillet, melt 1 teaspoon of coconut oil over medium heat and sauté onion for about 2-3 minutes.
4. Add the cabbage and stir fry for about 4-5 minutes.
5. Add the cooked apple slices, thyme and vinegar and cook, covered for about 1 minute.

6. Remove from the heat and serve warm.

# Herbed Asparagus

**Yield:** 4 servings

**Preparation Time:** 15 minutes

**Cooking Time:** 10 minutes

**Total Time:** 25 minutes

**Ingredients:**

- 2 tablespoons olive oil
- 2 tablespoons fresh lemon juice
- 1 tablespoon organic apple cider vinegar
- 1 teaspoon garlic, minced
- 1 tablespoon fresh parsley, chopped
- 1 teaspoon dried oregano
- Sea salt and freshly ground black pepper, to taste
- 1 pound fresh asparagus, ends removed

**Instructions:**

1. Preheat the oven to 400 degrees F. Lightly grease a rimmed baking sheet.
2. In a bowl, add the oil, lemon juice, vinegar, garlic, herbs, salt and black pepper and beat until well combined.
3. Arrange the asparagus onto the prepared baking sheet in a single layer.
4. Top with half of the herb mixture and toss to coat.
5. Roast for about 8-10 minutes.

6. Remove from the oven and transfer the asparagus onto a platter.

7. Drizzle with the remaining herb mixture and serve immediately.

# Veggie Kabobs

**Yield:** 4 servings

**Preparation Time:** 20 minutes

**Cooking Time:** 10 minutes

**Total Time:** 30 minutes

**Ingredients:**

**For Marinade:**

- 2 garlic cloves, minced
- 2 teaspoons fresh basil, minced
- 2 teaspoons fresh oregano, minced
- ½ teaspoon cayenne pepper
- Sea salt and freshly ground black pepper, to taste
- 2 tablespoons fresh lemon juice
- 2 tablespoons olive oil

**For Veggies:**

- 16 large button mushrooms, quartered
- 1 yellow bell pepper, seeded and cubed
- 1 red bell pepper, seeded and cubed
- 1 orange bell pepper, seeded and cubed
- 1 green bell pepper, seeded and cubed

**Instructions:**

1. For marinade: in a large bowl, add all the ingredients and mix until well combined.
2. Add the vegetables and toss to coat well.
3. Cover the bowl and refrigerate to marinate for at least 6-8 hours.
4. Preheat the grill to medium-high heat. Generously, grease the grill grate.
5. Remove the vegetables from the bowl and thread onto pre-soaked wooden skewers.
6. Place the skewers onto the grill and cook for about 8-10 minutes or until done completely, flipping occasionally.
7. Remove from the grill and serve hot.

# Tofu with Brussels Sprout

**Yield:** 4 servings

**Preparation Time:** 15 minutes

**Cooking Time:** 15 minutes

**Total Time:** 30 minutes

**Ingredients:**

- 1 tablespoon olive oil, divided
- 8 ounces extra-firm tofu, drained, pressed and cut into slices
- 2 garlic cloves, chopped
- 1/3 cup pecans, toasted and chopped
- 1 tablespoon unsweetened applesauce
- ¼ cup fresh parsley, chopped
- ½ pound Brussels sprouts, trimmed and cut into wide ribbons

**Instructions:**

1. In a skillet, heat ½ tablespoon of the oil over medium heat and sauté the tofu and for about 6-7 minutes or until golden brown.
2. Add the garlic and pecans and sauté for about 1 minute.
3. Add the applesauce and cook for about 2 minutes.
4. Stir in the parsley and remove from heat.

5. With a slotted spoon, transfer the tofu onto a plate and set aside

6. In the same skillet, heat the remaining oil over medium-high heat and cook the Brussels sprouts for about 5 minutes.

7. Stir in the cooked tofu and remove from the heat.

8. Serve immediately.

# Tofu with Broccoli

**Yield:** 3 servings

**Preparation Time:** 15 minutes

**Cooking Time:** 13 minutes

**Total Time:** 28 minutes

**Ingredients:**

- 1 (12-ounce) package firm tofu, drained, pressed, and cut into 5 slices
- 2 tablespoons coconut oil, divided
- 2 cups small broccoli florets
- ¼ cup alkaline water
- ½ tablespoon garlic, minced
- ½ tablespoon fresh ginger root, minced
- Sea salt and freshly ground black pepper, to taste

**Instructions:**

1. In a large non-stick skillet, melt 1 tablespoon of the coconut oil over medium-high heat and cook the tofu for 4-5 minutes per side or until crispy.
2. With a slotted spoon, scoop the tofu slices onto a paper towel-lined plate to absorb any extra oil.
3. Then, cut each tofu slice into equal-sized pieces.
4. Meanwhile, in a large microwave-safe bowl, add the broccoli florets and water.

5. Cover the bowl and microwave on High for about 5 minutes.

6. Remove from the microwave and drain the broccoli.

7. In the same skillet, melt the remaining coconut oil over medium heat and sauté the garlic and ginger for about 1 minute.

8. Add the tofu, broccoli and black pepper and cook for 2 minutes, tossing occasionally.

9. Remove from the heat and serve hot.

# Tempeh in Tomato Sauce

**Yield:** 4 servings

**Preparation Time:** 20 minutes

**Cooking Time:** 1 hour 20 minutes

**Total Time:** 1 hour 40 minutes

**Ingredients:**

- ½ cup extra-virgin oil, divided
- 2 (8-ounce) packages tempeh, cut into ½-inch slices horizontally
- 1 large yellow onion, chopped
- 3 garlic cloves, minced
- 1 teaspoon dried oregano, crushed
- 1 teaspoon dried thyme, crushed
- ½ teaspoon red chili powder
- ½ teaspoon red pepper flakes, crushed
- 1 large green bell pepper, seeded and sliced thinly
- 1 large yellow bell pepper, seeded and sliced thinly
- 2 cups fresh tomatoes, chopped finely
- ¼ cup homemade tomato paste
- 1 teaspoon organic apple cider vinegar
- 1 tablespoon maple syrup

**Instructions:**

1. Preheat the oven to 350 degrees F.

2. In a large bowl, add 2 tablespoons of oil and tempeh slices and toss to coat well.

3. In a large skillet, heat ¼ cup of oil over medium-high heat and cook the tempeh slices for about 5-7 minutes.

4. Carefully, change the side and cook for about 5-7 minutes.

5. Transfer the cooked tempeh slices onto a paper towel-lined plate.

6. Set aside to drain.

7. Meanwhile, in another non-stick skillet, heat the remaining oil over medium-low heat and sauté the onion, garlic, herbs and spices for about 8-10 minutes.

8. Add the bell peppers and sauté for about 4-5 minutes, stirring occasionally.

9. Add the remaining ingredients and stir until well combined.

10. Remove from the heat.

11. In the bottom of a large casserole dish, arrange the tempeh slices.

12. Place the tomato mixture over tempeh slices evenly.

13. With a piece of foil, cover the casserole dish tightly.

14. Bake for about 1 hour.

15. Remove from the oven and set aside to cool slightly.

16. Serve warm.

# Salad Recipes

## Apple & Strawberry Salad

**Yield:** 4 servings

**Preparation Time:** 15 minutes

**Total Time:** 15 minutes

**Ingredients:**

**For Salad:**

- 2 apples, cored and sliced
- 1 cup fresh strawberries, hulled and sliced
- ¼ cup pecans, toasted and chopped
- 4 cups mixed lettuce, torn

**For Dressing:**

- 3 tablespoons organic apple cider vinegar
- 3 tablespoons extra-virgin olive oil
- 1 tablespoon agave nectar
- Sea salt and freshly ground black pepper, to taste

**Instructions:**

1. For salad: in a large bowl, place all the ingredients and mix well.
2. For dressing: in another bowl, place all the ingredients in a bowl and beat until well combined.

3.  Pour the dressing over salad and gently, toss to coat well.

4.  Serve immediately.

# Mixed Berries Salad

**Yield:** 6 servings

**Preparation Time:** 15 minutes

**Total Time:** 15 minutes

**Ingredients:**

- 1 cup fresh strawberries, hulled and sliced
- 1 cup fresh blackberries
- 1 cup fresh raspberries
- 6 cups fresh rocket
- 3 tablespoons extra-virgin olive oil
- Sea salt and freshly ground black pepper, to taste

**Instructions:**

1. In a large bowl, place all the ingredients and gently, toss to coat well.
2. Serve immediately.

# Raspberry & Walnut Salad

**Yield:** 2 servings

**Preparation Time:** 15 minutes

**Total Time:** 15 minutes

**Ingredients:**

**For Salad:**

- 3 cups fresh baby kale
- 1 cup fresh raspberries
- ¼ cup walnuts, chopped

**For Dressing:**

- 1 tablespoon extra-virgin olive oil
- 1 tablespoon apple cider vinegar
- ½ teaspoon pure maple syrup
- Sea salt and freshly ground black pepper, to taste

**Instructions:**

1. For salad: in a large bowl, place all the ingredients and mix well.
2. For dressing: in another bowl, place all the ingredients in a bowl and beat until well combined.
3. Pour the dressing over salad and gently, toss to coat well.
4. Serve immediately.

# Orange & Grapefruit Salad

**Yield:** 2 servings

**Preparation Time:** 15 minutes

**Total Time:** 15 minutes

**Ingredients:**

**For Salad:**

- 3 cups fresh kale, tough ribs removed and torn
- 1 orange, peeled and segmented
- 1 grapefruit, peeled and segmented

**For Dressing:**

- 2 tablespoons extra-virgin olive oil
- 2 tablespoons fresh orange juice
- 1 teaspoon Dijon mustard
- ½ teaspoon agave nectar
- Sea salt and freshly ground black pepper, to taste

**Instructions:**

1. For salad: in a large bowl, place all the ingredients and mix well.
2. For dressing: in another bowl, place all the ingredients in a bowl and beat until well combined.
3. Pour the dressing over salad and gently, toss to coat well.
4. Serve immediately.

# Mango, Papaya & Pineapple Salad

**Yield:** 2 servings

**Preparation Time:** 15 minutes

**Total Time:** 15 minutes

**Ingredients:**

**For Salad:**

- 3 cups fresh baby kale
- ½ cup mango, peeled, pitted and cubed
- ½ cup fresh papaya, peeled, seeded and cubed
- ½ cup fresh pineapple, peeled and cubed
- ¼ cup almonds, chopped

**For Dressing:**

- 2 tablespoons extra-virgin olive oil
- 3 tablespoons fresh lime juice
- 2 tablespoons maple syrup
- Sea salt and freshly ground black pepper, to taste

**Instructions:**

1. For salad: in a large bowl, place all the ingredients and mix well.
2. For dressing: in another bowl, place all the ingredients in a bowl and beat until well combined.

3.  Pour the dressing over salad and gently, toss to coat well.

4.  Serve immediately.

# Mango & Avocado Salad

**Yield:** 6 servings

**Preparation Time:** 15 minutes

**Total Time:** 15 minutes

**Ingredients:**

- 2½ cups mango, peeled, pitted and sliced
- 2½ cups avocado, peeled, pitted and sliced
- 1 red onion, sliced
- 6 cups fresh baby arugula
- ¼ cup fresh mint leaves, chopped
- 2 tablespoon fresh orange juice
- Sea salt, to taste

**Instructions:**

1. In a large serving bowl, place all the ingredients and gently, toss to coat.
2. Cover the bowl and refrigerate to chill before serving.

# Cabbage & Carrot Salad

**Yield:** 5 servings

**Preparation Time:** 15 minutes

**Total Time:** 15 minutes

**Ingredients:**

- 2 cups purple cabbage, shredded
- 2 cups green cabbage, shredded
- 2 cups carrot, peeled and chopped
- 2 large scallions, chopped
- ¼ cup fresh parsley leaves, chopped
- 1 jalapeño pepper, seeded and minced
- 2 tablespoons fresh lemon juice
- 2 tablespoons extra-virgin olive oil
- Sea salt and freshly ground black pepper, to taste
- 2 tablespoons walnuts, chopped
- 1 teaspoon fresh lemon zest, grated finely

**Instructions:**

1. In a large serving bowl, add all the ingredients except lemon zest and toss to coat well.
2. Serve immediately with the garnishing of walnuts and lemon zest.

# Cucumber & Tomato Salad

**Yield:** 4 servings

**Preparation Time:** 15 minutes

**Total Time:** 15 minutes

**Ingredients:**

- 2 cups cucumbers, chopped
- 1 cup red grape tomatoes, halved
- 1 cup yellow grape tomatoes, halved
- 2 cups mixed fresh lettuce, torn
- 2 cups fresh baby kale
- 2 tablespoons extra-virgin olive oil
- 2 tablespoons fresh lime juice
- Sea salt, to taste

**Instructions:**

1. In a large serving bowl, add all the ingredients except lemon zest and toss to coat well.
2. Serve immediately.

# Mixed Veggies & Avocado Salad

**Yield:** 8 servings

**Preparation Time:** 20 minutes

**Total Time:** 20 minutes

**Ingredients:**

**For Dressing:**

- 1/3 cup extra-virgin olive oil
- ½ cup fresh lemon juice
- 1 tablespoon fresh ginger, grated
- 2 teaspoons Dijon mustard
- 2 teaspoons pure maple syrup
- Sea salt, to taste

**For Salad:**

- 2 large avocados, peeled, pitted and chopped
- 2 tablespoons fresh lemon juice
- 2 cups fresh baby kale, sliced thinly
- 2 cups small broccoli florets
- 1 cup red cabbage, shredded
- 1 cup purple cabbage, shredded
- 2 large carrots, peeled and grated
- 1 small orange bell pepper, seeded and sliced into matchsticks

- 1 small yellow bell pepper, seeded and sliced into matchsticks
- ½ cup fresh parsley leaves, chopped
- 1 cup walnuts, chopped

## Instructions:

1. For dressing: in a food processor, add all the ingredients and pulse until well combined and smooth.
2. For salad: in a bowl, add the avocado slices and lime juice and toss to coat well.
3. Add the remaining vegetables and toss to coat well.
4. Top with walnuts and serve immediately.

# Mixed Veggie Noodles Salad

**Yield:** 8 servings

**Preparation Time:** 20 minutes

**Total Time:** 20 minutes

**Ingredients:**

**For Salad:**

- 3 large zucchinis, spiralized with Blade C
- 2 large yellow squashes, spiralized with Blade C
- 2 carrots, peeled and spiralized with Blade C
- 2 cups grape tomatoes, halved
- 1/3 cup olive oil

**For Pesto:**

- 2 cups fresh basil leaves
- 1 cup fresh parsley leaves
- ½ cup pine nuts
- 1 garlic clove, peeled
- ½ cup olive oil
- 1 tablespoon fresh lemon juice
- Sea salt and freshly ground black pepper, to taste

**Instructions:**

1. For salad: in a large bowl, add vegetable noodles, tomatoes and oil, and toss to coat well.

2. For pesto: in a food processor, add all ingredients and pulse until smooth.
3. Place the pesto over salad and gently, stir to combine.
4. Serve immediately.

# Quinoa & Mango Salad

**Yield:** 4 servings

**Preparation Time:** 15 minutes

**Cooking Time:** 20 minutes

**Total Time:** 35 minutes

**Ingredients:**

- ¾ cup red quinoa, rinsed and drained
- ¼ teaspoon garlic powder
- ¼ teaspoon ground cumin
- Sea salt and freshly ground black pepper, to taste
- 1½ cups homemade vegetable broth
- 1 large mango, peeled, pitted and cubed
- 3 scallions, chopped

**Instructions:**

1. In a pan, add the quinoa, garlic powder, cumin, salt, black pepper and broth over high heat and bring to a boil.
2. Reduce the heat to medium-low and simmer, covered for about 15-20 minutes or until all the liquid is absorbed.
3. Remove from the heat and set aside, covered for about 5 minutes.
4. Uncover the pan and with a fork, fluff the quinoa.
5. Set aside to cool completely.
6. Transfer the quinoa into a large bowl.

7. Add the remaining ingredients and stir to combine.

8. Serve immediately.

# Chickpeas, Lentils & Veggie Salad

**Yield:** 6 servings

**Preparation Time:** 15 minutes

**Cooking Time:** 35 minutes

**Total Time:** 50 minutes

**Ingredients:**

- 1½ cups alkaline water
- ½ cup dry red lentils
- 1 (15-ounce) can low-sodium chickpeas, rinsed and drained
- 1 green bell pepper, seeded and chopped
- 1 yellow bell pepper, seeded and chopped
- 1 red bell pepper, seeded and chopped
- 2 large tomatoes, chopped
- 4 scallions, chopped
- 2 jalapeño peppers, minced
- 2 tablespoon olive oil
- 2 tablespoons fresh lime juice
- Sea salt, to taste
- ¼ cup fresh parsley, chopped

**Instructions:**

1. In a large pan, add the water and lentils over high heat and bring to a boil.

2. Reduce the heat to low and simmer, covered for about 30 minutes or until all the liquid is absorbed and lentils become tender.

3. Transfer the lentils into a large bowl and set aside to cool completely.

4. After cooling, add the remaining all ingredients and toss to coat well.

5. Serve immediately.

# Beans, Papaya & Avocado Salad

**Yield:** 6 servings

**Preparation Time:** 15 minutes

**Total Time:** 15 minutes

**Ingredients:**

**For Salad:**

- 3 cups cooked black beans, drained
- 2 cups papaya, peeled and cubed
- 1 medium ripe avocado, peeled, pitted and cubed
- 2 Serrano peppers, seeded and chopped finely
- ¼ cup fresh parsley, minced

**For Dressing:**

- 2 garlic cloves, minced
- 1 tablespoon organic apple cider vinegar
- ¼ cup fresh orange juice
- 2 tablespoons fresh lime juice
- 2-3 drops liquid stevia
- ¼ teaspoon red chili pepper
- Sea salt, to taste

**Instructions:**

1. For salad: in a large bowl, place all the ingredients and mix well.

2. For dressing: in another bowl, place all the ingredients in a bowl and beat until well combined.

3. Pour the dressing over salad and gently, toss to coat well.

4. Serve immediately.

# Herbed Beans Salad

**Yield:** 4 servings

**Preparation Time:** 15 minutes

**Total Time:** 15 minutes

**Ingredients:**

**For Salad:**

- 2 cups fresh green beans, trimmed and halved
- 1 (15-ounce) can low-sodium red kidney beans, rinsed and drained
- 1 (15-ounce) can low-sodium cannellini beans, rinsed and drained
- ¼ cup fresh parsley leaves, chopped
- ¼ cup fresh basil leaves, chopped

**For Dressing:**

- 1 shallot, minced
- ½ cup extra-virgin olive oil
- ¼ cup organic apple cider vinegar
- 1 tablespoon maple syrup
- 2 teaspoons Dijon mustard
- Sea salt and freshly ground black pepper, to taste

## Instructions:

1. In a large pan of the salted boiling water, add the green beans and cook for about 2-3 minutes.
2. Drain the green beans well and transfer into a bowl of chilled water.
3. Again, drain the green beans well and transfer into a large bowl.
4. In the bowl of green beans, add the remaining salad ingredients and mix.
5. For dressing: in another bowl, place all the ingredients in a bowl and beat until well combined.
6. Pour the dressing over salad and gently, toss to coat well.
7. Serve immediately.

# Mixed Beans Salad

**Yield:** 8 servings

**Preparation Time:** 15 minutes

**Total Time:** 15 minutes

**Ingredients:**

**For Salad:**

- 1¼ cups cooked cannellini beans
- 1¼ cups cooked red kidney beans
- 1¼ cups cooked black beans
- 1¼ cups cooked garbanzo beans
- 2 cups cucumber, chopped
- 1 cup red onion, chopped
- 1½ cups plum tomato, chopped

**For Dressing:**

- 1 garlic clove, minced
- 2 tablespoons shallots, minced
- 2 teaspoons lemon zest, grated finely
- ¼ cup fresh lime juice
- 2 tablespoons extra-virgin olive oil
- Sea salt and freshly ground black pepper, to taste

**Instructions:**

1. For salad: in a large bowl, place all the ingredients and mix well.
2. For dressing: in another bowl, place all the ingredients in a bowl and beat until well combined.
3. Pour the dressing over salad and gently, toss to coat well.
4. Serve immediately.

# Snack Recipes

## Grilled Watermelon

**Yield:** 4 servings

**Preparation Time:** 10 minutes

**Cooking Time:** 4 minutes

**Total Time:** 14 minutes

**Ingredients:**

- 1 medium watermelon, peeled and cut into 1-inch thick wedges
- 1 garlic clove, minced finely
- 2 tablespoons fresh lime juice
- Pinch of cayenne pepper
- Pinch of sea salt

**Instructions:**

1. Preheat the grill to high heat. Grease the grill grate.
2. Place the watermelon wedges onto the grill and cook for about 2 minutes from both sides.
3. Meanwhile, in a small bowl mix together all ingredients.
4. Drizzle the watermelon slices with lemon mixture and serve.

# Kale Chips

**Yield:** 6 servings

**Preparation Time:** 10 minutes

**Cooking Time:** 15 minutes

**Total Time:** 25 minutes

**Ingredients:**

- 1 pound fresh kale leaves, tough ribs removed and torn
- ¼ teaspoon cayenne pepper
- Sea salt, to taste
- 1 tablespoon olive oil

**Instructions:**

1. Preheat the oven to 350 degrees F. Line a large baking sheet with parchment paper.
2. Arrange the kale pieces onto the prepared baking sheet in a single layer.
3. Sprinkle the kale with cayenne pepper and salt and drizzle with oil.
4. Bake for 10-15 minutes.
5. Remove from the oven and set aside to cool before serving.

# Strawberry Gazpacho

**Yield:** 4 servings

**Preparation Time:** 15 minutes

**Total Time:** 15 minutes

**Ingredients:**

- 1½ pounds fresh strawberries, hulled and sliced
- ½ cup red bell pepper, seeded and chopped
- 1 small cucumber, peeled, seeded and chopped
- ¼ cup red onion, chopped
- ¼ cup fresh basil leaves
- 1 small garlic clove, chopped
- ¼ of small jalapeño pepper, seeded and chopped
- 1 tablespoon olive oil
- 3 tablespoons organic apple cider vinegar

**Instructions:**

1. In a blender, add all the ingredients and pulse until smooth.
2. Transfer the gazpacho into a large bowl.
3. Cover the bowl and refrigerate to chill completely before serving.

# Mango & Avocado Salsa

**Yield:** 6 servings

**Preparation Time:** 15 minutes

**Total Time:** 15 minutes

**Ingredients:**

- 1 avocado, peeled, pitted and cut into cubes
- 2 tablespoons fresh lime juice
- 1 mango, peeled, pitted and cubed
- 1 cup cherry tomatoes, halved
- 1 jalapeño pepper, seeded and chopped
- 1 tablespoon fresh parsley, chopped
- Sea salt, to taste

**Instructions:**

1. In a large bowl, add and lime juice and mix well.
2. Add the remaining ingredients and stir to combine.
3. Serve immediately.

# Avocado Guacamole

**Yield:** 4 servings

**Preparation Time:** 10 minutes

**Total Time:** 10 minutes

**Ingredients:**

- 2 medium ripe avocados, peeled, pitted, and chopped
- 1 small red onion, chopped
- 1 garlic clove, minced
- 1 Serrano pepper, seeded and chopped
- 1 tomato, seeded and chopped
- 2 tablespoons fresh parsley leaves, chopped
- 1 tablespoon fresh lime juice
- Sea salt, to taste

**Instructions:**

1. In a large bowl, place the avocado and with a fork, mash it completely.
2. Add the remaining ingredients and gently stir to combine.
3. Serve immediately.

# Chickpeas Hummus

**Yield:** 12 servings

**Preparation Time:** 10 minutes

**Total Time:** 10 minutes

**Ingredients:**

- 2 (15-ounce) cans low-sodium chickpeas, rinsed and drained
- ½ cup tahini
- 1 garlic clove, chopped
- 2 tablespoons fresh lemon juice
- Sea salt, to taste
- Alkaline water, as needed
- 1 tablespoon olive oil
- Pinch of cayenne pepper

**Instructions:**

1. In a blender, add all the ingredients except the oil and cayenne pepper and pulse until smooth.
2. Transfer the hummus into a large bowl and drizzle with oil.
3. Sprinkle with cayenne pepper and serve immediately.

# Cauliflower Hummus

**Yield:** 6 servings

**Preparation Time:** 15 minutes

**Cooking Time:** 5 minutes

**Total Time:** 20 minutes

**Ingredients:**

- 1 medium head cauliflower, trimmed and chopped
- 2 garlic cloves, chopped
- 2 tablespoons almond butter
- 2 tablespoons olive oil
- Sea salt, to taste
- 2 tablespoons fresh chives, minced
- Pinch of cayenne pepper

**Instructions:**

1. In a large pan of the boiling water, add the cauliflower and bring to a boil.
2. Reduce the heat to medium and cook for about 4-5 minutes.
3. Remove from the heat and drain the cauliflower well.
4. Set aside to cool slightly.
5. In a food processor, add the cauliflower, garlic, almond butter, oil, and salt and pulse until smooth.
6. Transfer the hummus into a serving bowl.

7.  Sprinkle with chives and cayenne pepper and serve
    immediately.

# Spicy Veggie Bites

**Yield:** 6 servings

**Preparation Time:** 15 minutes

**Cooking Time:** 25 minutes

**Total Time:** 40 minutes

**Ingredients:**

- 2 medium sweet potatoes, peeled and cubed into ½-inch pieces
- 2 tablespoons unsweetened coconut milk
- 1 cup fresh kale leaves, tough ribs removed and chopped
- 1 medium shallot, chopped finely
- 1 teaspoon ground cumin
- ¼ teaspoon ground turmeric
- Sea salt and freshly ground black pepper, to taste

**Instructions:**

1. Preheat the oven to 400 degrees F. Line a baking sheet with parchment paper.
2. In a pan of the water, arrange a steamer basket.
3. Place the sweet potato cubes in the steamer basket and steam for about 10-15 minutes.
4. In a large bowl, add the sweet potatoes and coconut milk and with a potato masher, mash well.

5.  Add the remaining ingredients and mix until well combined.

6.  Make about 1½-2-inch balls from the mixture.

7.  Coat the veggie balls with

8.  Arrange the balls onto prepared baking sheet in a single layer.

9.  Bake for about 20-25 minutes.

10. Remove from the oven and set the balls aside to cool slightly.

11. Serve warm.

# Sweet & Savory Fennel Cookies

**Yield:** 6 servings

**Preparation Time:** 15 minutes

**Cooking Time:** 9 minutes

**Total Time:** 24 minutes

**Ingredients:**

- 1/3 cup coconut flour
- ¼ teaspoon whole fennel seeds
- Pinch of ground cinnamon
- Pinch of ground cardamom
- Pinch of ground cloves
- Pinch of sea salt
- Pinch of freshly ground black pepper
- ¼ cup coconut oil, softened
- 2 tablespoons maple syrup
- 1 teaspoon organic vanilla extract
- ½ teaspoon fresh ginger root, peeled and grated finely

**Instructions:**

1. Preheat the oven to 360 degrees F. Line a cookie sheet with parchment paper.
2. In a large bowl, add the flour, fennel seeds, spices, salt, and black pepper and mix well.

3. In another bowl, add the coconut oil, maple syrup, and vanilla extract and beat until well combined.

4. Add the ginger and stir to combine.

5. Add the flour mixture and mix until a smooth dough forms.

6. Make small, equal-sized balls from the mixture.

7. Arrange the balls onto the prepared cookie sheet about 1-inch apart in a single layer and, with your fingers, gently press down each ball to form the cookies.

8. Bake for about 9 minutes or until golden brown.

9. Remove from the oven and place the cookie sheet onto a wire rack to cool in the pan for about 5 minutes.

10. Carefully, invert the cookies onto the wire rack to cool completely before serving.

# Seeds Crackers

**Yield:** 6 servings

**Preparation Time:** 15 minutes

**Cooking Time:** 20 minutes

**Total Time:** 35 minutes

**Ingredients:**

- 1 tablespoon chia seeds
- 3 tablespoons alkaline water
- 3 tablespoons sunflower seeds
- 1 tablespoon quinoa flour
- 1 teaspoon ground turmeric
- Pinch of ground cinnamon
- Sea salt, to taste

**Instructions:**

1. Preheat the oven to 345 degrees F. Line a baking sheet with parchment paper.
2. In a large bowl, add the chia seeds and water and stir to combine.
3. Set aside for about 15 minutes.
4. After 15 minutes, add the remaining ingredients and mix well.
5. Spread the mixture onto the prepared baking sheet and with the back of a spoon, smooth the top surface.

6.  With a pizza slicer, slice into desired shapes.

7.  Bake for about 20 minutes.

8.  Remove from the oven and place onto a wire rack to cool completely before serving.

# Soup Recipes

## Basil Tomato Soup

**Yield:** 4 servings

**Preparation Time:** 10 minutes

**Cooking Time:** 45 minutes

**Total Time:** 55 minutes

**Ingredients:**

- 2 tablespoons coconut oil
- 2 carrots, peeled and chopped roughly
- 1 large white onion, chopped roughly
- 3 garlic cloves, minced
- 5 large tomatoes, chopped roughly
- ¼ cup fresh basil, chopped
- 1 tablespoon homemade tomato paste
- 3 cups homemade vegetable broth
- ¼ cup unsweetened coconut milk
- Sea salt and freshly ground black pepper, to taste

**Instructions:**

1. In a large pan, melt the coconut oil over medium heat and cook the carrot and onion for about 10 minutes, stirring frequently.
2. Add the garlic and sauté for 1-2 minutes.

3. Stir in the tomatoes, basil, tomato paste, and broth and bring to a boil.

4. Reduce the heat to low and simmer for about 30 minutes.

5. Stir in the coconut milk, salt, and black pepper and remove from the heat.

6. With an immersion blender, blend the soup until smooth.

7. Serve hot.

# Broccoli Soup

**Yield:** 4 servings

**Preparation Time:** 15 minutes

**Cooking Time:** 45 minutes

**Total Time:** 1 hour

**Ingredients:**

- 2 tablespoons olive oil
- ½ cup onion, chopped
- 1 garlic clove, minced
- 1 tablespoon fresh thyme, chopped
- ¼ teaspoon ground cumin
- ¼ teaspoon red pepper flakes, crushed
- 2 medium heads broccoli, cut into florets
- 4 cups homemade vegetable broth
- 1 avocado, peeled, pitted and chopped

**Instructions:**

1. In a large soup pan, heat the oil over medium heat and sauté the onion for about 4-5 minutes.
2. Add the garlic, thyme and spices and sauté for about 1 minute more.
3. Add the broccoli and cook for about 3-4 minutes.
4. Add the broth and stir to combine.
5. Increase the heat to high and bring to a boil.

6.  Reduce the heat to medium-low and simmer, covered for about 32-35 minutes.

7.  Remove from the heat and set aside to cool slightly.

8.  In a blender, place the mixture in batches with avocado and pulse until smooth.

9.  Serve immediately.

# Cauliflower Soup

**Yield:** 4 servings

**Preparation Time:** 15 minutes

**Cooking Time:** 25 minutes

**Total Time:** 40 minutes

**Ingredients:**

- 2 tablespoons olive oil
- 1 large yellow onion, chopped
- 2 large carrots, peeled and chopped
- 2 garlic cloves, minced
- 1 Serrano pepper, chopped finely
- 1 teaspoon ground turmeric
- 1 teaspoon ground coriander
- 1 teaspoon ground cumin
- ¼ teaspoon red pepper flakes, crushed
- 1 head cauliflower, chopped
- 4 cups homemade vegetable broth
- 1 cup unsweetened coconut milk
- Sea salt and freshly ground black pepper, to taste
- 2 tablespoons fresh chives, chopped

**Instructions:**

1. In a large pan, heat the oil over medium heat and sauté the onion and carrot for 5-6 minutes.

2. Add the garlic, Serrano pepper and spices and sauté for about 1 minute.

3. Add the cauliflower and cook for 5 minutes, stirring occasionally.

4. Add the broth and coconut milk and bring to a boil over medium-high heat.

5. Reduce the heat to low and simmer for 15 minutes.

6. Season the soup with salt and black pepper and remove from the heat.

7. Serve hot with a garnishing of chives.

# Pumpkin Soup

**Yield:** 4 servings

**Preparation Time:** 15 minutes

**Cooking Time:** 25 minutes

**Total Time:** 40 minutes

**Ingredients:**

- 2 teaspoons olive oil
- 1 onion, chopped
- 1 teaspoon fresh ginger, chopped
- 2 garlic cloves, chopped
- 2 tablespoons fresh parsley, chopped
- 3 cups pumpkin, peeled and cubed
- 4¼ cups homemade vegetable broth
- Sea salt and freshly ground black pepper, to taste
- ½ cup coconut cream
- 2 tablespoons fresh lime juice

**Instructions:**

1. In a large soup pan, heat oil over medium heat and sauté the onion, turmeric, ginger, garlic and parsley for about 3-4 minutes.
2. Add the pumpkin and broth and bring to a boil
3. Reduce the heat to low and simmer, covered for about 15 minutes.

4. Remove from heat and set aside to cool slightly.

5. Transfer the mixture into a high-speed blender in batches with avocado and pulse until smooth.

6. Return the soup into the pan over medium heat and cook for 3 minutes or until heated through.

7. Serve hot.

# Asparagus Soup

**Yield:** 4 servings

**Preparation Time:** 15 minutes

**Cooking Time:** 40 minutes

**Total Time:** 55 minutes

**Ingredients:**

- 1 tablespoon olive oil
- 3 scallions, chopped
- 1½ pounds fresh asparagus, trimmed and chopped
- 4 cups homemade vegetable broth
- 2 tablespoons fresh lemon juice
- Sea salt and freshly ground black pepper, to taste
- 2 tablespoons coconut cream

**Instructions:**

1. In a large pan, heat the oil over medium heat and sauté the scallion for 2 minutes.
2. Stir in the asparagus and broth and bring to a boil.
3. Reduce the heat to low and simmer, covered for 25-30 minutes.
4. Remove from the heat and set aside to cool slightly.
5. Now, transfer the soup into a high-speed blender in 2 batches and pulse until smooth.

6. Return the soup into the same pan over medium heat and simmer for 4-5 minutes.

7. Stir in the lemon juice, salt, and black pepper and remove from the heat.

8. Serve hot with a topping of coconut cream.

# Mushroom Soup

**Yield:** 5 servings

**Preparation Time:** 15 minutes

**Cooking Time:** 20 minutes

**Total Time:** 35 minutes

**Ingredients:**

- 2 teaspoons olive oil
- 1 large yellow onion, chopped
- 2 medium carrots, peeled and chopped
- 2 garlic cloves, minced
- 6 cups homemade vegetable broth
- 1 pound fresh button mushrooms, sliced thinly
- 2 scallions, chopped
- Sea salt and freshly ground black pepper, to taste

**Instructions:**

1. In a large pan, heat the oil over medium heat and sauté onion, carrot and garlic for about 4-5 minutes.
2. Add the broth and bring to a boil.
3. Cook for about 1-2 minutes.
4. Add the mushrooms and bring to a boil.
5. Cook for about 7-8 minutes.
6. Stir in scallions, salt and black pepper and cook for about 2 minutes.

7.  Serve hot.

# Carrot Soup

**Yield:** 4 servings

**Preparation Time:** 15 minutes

**Cooking Time:** 35 minutes

**Total Time:** 50 minutes

**Ingredients:**

- 2 tablespoons olive oil
- 1 large yellow onion, chopped
- 2 large garlic cloves, minced
- 1 Serrano pepper, chopped finely
- 4 large carrots, peeled and chopped
- 4 cups homemade vegetable broth
- 2 tablespoons fresh parsley, chopped
- 2 tablespoons fresh lime juice
- Sea salt and freshly ground black pepper, to taste
- 1 teaspoon fresh lime zest, grated finely

**Instructions:**

1. In a large soup pan, heat the oil over medium heat and sauté the onion for about 4-5 minutes.
2. Add the garlic and Serrano pepper and sauté for about 1 minute.
3. Add the carrots and cook for about 3-4 minutes, stirring occasionally.

4.  Add the broth and stir to combine.

5.  Increase the heat to medium-high and bring to a boil.

6.  Reduce the heat to medium-low and simmer for about 20 minutes.

7.  Remove from the heat and with an immersion blender, blend the soup until smooth.

8.  Return the pan over medium heat.

9.  Cook for about 2-3 minutes.

10. Stir in the parsley, lime juice, salt and black pepper and remove from the heat.

11. Serve hot with the topping of lime zest.

# Squash & Apple Soup

**Yield:** 4 servings

**Preparation Time:** 15 minutes

**Cooking Time:** 45 minutes

**Total Time:** 1 hour

**Ingredients:**

- 2 tablespoon extra-virgin olive oil
- 1 cup white onion, chopped
- 2 garlic cloves, minced
- 1 teaspoon dried thyme
- 3 cups butternut squash, peeled, seeded and chopped
- 2 apple, cored and chopped
- 4 cups homemade vegetable broth
- Sea salt, to taste

**Instructions:**

1. In a large pan, heat the oil over medium heat and sauté the onion for about 5 minutes.
2. Add the garlic and thyme and sauté for about 1 minute.
3. Add the squash, apple and ginger and cook for about 1-2 minutes.
4. Stir in the broth and bring to a boil.
5. Reduce the heat to low and simmer covered for about 30 minutes.

6. Stir in the salt and remove from the heat.

7. With an immersion blender, blend the soup until smooth.

8. Serve immediately.

# Green Veggies Soup

**Yield:** 8 servings

**Preparation Time:** 20 minutes

**Cooking Time:** 5 minutes

**Total Time:** 25 minutes

**Ingredients:**

- ¼ cup almonds, soaked overnight and drained
- 1 large avocado, peeled, pitted and chopped
- ½ of green bell pepper, seeded and chopped
- 2 cups fresh spinach leaves
- 1 small zucchini, chopped
- 1 large celery stalk, chopped
- 2 tablespoons yellow onion, chopped
- 1 garlic clove, chopped
- ½ cup fresh parsley leaves
- ¼ cup fresh basil leaves
- 2 tablespoons fresh lemon juice
- Sea salt and freshly ground black pepper, to taste
- 2 cups homemade vegetable broth

**Instructions:**

1. In a high-speed blender, add all ingredients and pulse until smooth.

2. Transfer the soup into a pan over medium heat and cook
   for about 4-5 minutes or until heated through.
3. Remove from the heat and serve immediately.

# Mixed Veggies Soup

**Yield:** 8 servings

**Preparation Time:** 15 minutes

**Cooking Time:** 50 minutes

**Total Time:** 1 hour 5 minutes

**Ingredients:**

- 2 tablespoons olive oil
- 1 medium yellow onion, chopped
- 2 carrots, peeled and chopped
- 2 bay leaves
- ½ teaspoon ground cumin
- ½ teaspoon red chili powder
- ½ teaspoon smoked paprika
- 1 teaspoon garlic powder
- 2 cups fresh tomatoes, chopped finely
- 3 cups small cauliflower florets
- 3 cups small broccoli florets
- 8 cups homemade vegetable broth
- 4 cups fresh spinach, chopped
- 3 tablespoons fresh lemon juice
- Sea salt and freshly ground black pepper, to taste

**Instructions:**

1.  In a large soup pan, heat the oil over medium heat and sauté the onion, celery and carrot for about 5-6 minutes.
2.  Add the bay leaves and spices and sauté for about 1 minute.
3.  Add the tomatoes and cook for about 2-3 minutes, crushing with the back of a spoon.
4.  Add the cauliflower, broccoli and broth and bring to a boil on high heat.
5.  Reduce the heat to low. Cover and simmer for about 20-25 minutes.
6.  Stir in the spinach simmer for about 10 minutes more.
7.  Stir in lemon juice, salt and black pepper and remove from heat.
8.  Discard bay leaves and serve hot.

# Roasted Veggies Soup

**Yield:** 5 servings

**Preparation Time:** 20 minutes

**Cooking Time:** 1¼ hours

**Total Time:** 1 hour 35 minutes

**Ingredients:**

- 2 medium red bell peppers, halved and seeded
- ½ head of cauliflower, cut into florets
- ¼ cup olive oil, divided
- Sea salt and freshly ground black pepper, to taste
- 3 scallions, chopped
- 1 teaspoon dried thyme, crushed
- 1 teaspoon dried rosemary, crushed
- 1 teaspoon garlic powder
- 1 teaspoon ground cumin
- 1 teaspoon smoked paprika
- ¼ teaspoon red pepper flakes, crushed
- 4 cups homemade vegetable broth
- ½ cup coconut cream
- ¼ cup fresh parsley leaves, chopped

**Instructions:**

1. Preheat the broiler of oven. Line a baking sheet with a piece of foil.

2.  Arrange the bell peppers onto the prepared baking sheet, skin side up.

3.  Broil for about 10-15 minutes.

4.  Remove from the oven and immediately, transfer the peppers into an airtight container.

5.  Immediately, cover the container tightly and set aside for about 15-20 minutes.

6.  Now, set the temperature of the oven to 400 degrees F. Line a large baking sheet with a piece of foil.

7.  In a bowl, add the cauliflower florets, 2 tablespoons of the oil, salt and black pepper and toss to coat well.

8.  Arrange the cauliflower florets onto the prepared baking sheet in a single layer.

9.  Roast for about 30-35 minutes, tossing twice.

10. Meanwhile, remove the bell peppers from the container and carefully, peel the skin.

11. Then, chop each bell pepper roughly and transfer into a bowl.

12. Remove the cauliflower florets from the oven and transfer into the bowl of bell peppers.

13. In a large pan, heat the remaining oil over medium heat and sauté the scallions for about 2-3 minutes.

14. Add the thyme, rosemary and spices and sauté for about 1 minute.

15. Add the broth, bell peppers and cauliflower and bring to a boil.

16. Reduce the heat to medium-low and simmer for about 15-20 minutes.
17. With an immersion blender, blend the mixture until smooth finely.
18. Stir in the coconut cream, salt and black pepper and remove from the heat.
19. Serve hot with the garnishing of parsley.

# Tofu & Veggies Soup

**Yield:** 4 servings

**Preparation Time:** 20 minutes

**Cooking Time:** 15 minutes

**Total Time:** 35 minutes

**Ingredients:**

- 1 tablespoon olive oil
- 1 garlic clove, minced
- ½ teaspoon fresh ginger, minced
- 1 lemongrass stalk, chopped finely
- Pinch of red pepper flakes, crushed
- ¼ cup fresh mushrooms, sliced
- 2 cups alkaline water
- 2 cups homemade vegetable broth
- 1 large zucchini, peeled and spiralized with Blade C
- 2 cups baby bok choy, trimmed and chopped
- ¼ cup scallions, chopped
- ½ cup tofu, drained, pressed and cubed
- 1 tablespoon fresh lime juice
- Sea salt and freshly ground black pepper, to taste
- 2 tablespoons fresh parsley, chopped

**Instructions:**

1. In a large soup pan, heat the oil over medium heat and sauté the garlic, ginger, lemongrass and red pepper flakes for about 2 minutes.
2. Add the mushrooms and cook for about 3-4 minutes.
3. Add the water and broth and stir to combine.
4. Increase the heat to high and bring to a boil.
5. Add the zucchini, bok choy, scallions, tofu, lime juice and stir to combine.
6. Reduced the heat to medium and cook for about 4-5 minutes.
7. Stir in the salt and black pepper and remove from the heat.
8. Garnish with parsley and serve hot.

# Lentils & Veggie Soup

**Yield:** 8 servings

**Preparation Time:** 15 minutes

**Cooking Time:** 1¼ hours

**Total Time:** 1½ hours

**Ingredients:**

- 2 tablespoons olive oil
- 3 carrots, peeled and chopped
- 2 sweet onions, chopped
- 3 garlic cloves, minced
- 1¾ cups brown lentils, rinsed
- 2½ cups tomatoes, chopped finely
- ¼ teaspoon dried basil, crushed
- ¼ teaspoon dried oregano, crushed
- ¼ teaspoon dried thyme, crushed
- 1 teaspoon ground cumin
- ½ teaspoon ground coriander
- ½ teaspoon paprika
- 6 cups homemade vegetable broth
- 3 cups fresh collard greens, chopped
- Sea salt and freshly ground black pepper, to taste
- 2 tablespoons fresh lemon juice

**Instructions:**

1. In a large soup pan, heat the oil over medium heat and sauté carrot and onion for 5 minutes.
2. Add the garlic, sauté for about 1 minute.
3. Add the lentils and sauté for 3 minutes.
4. Stir in the tomatoes, herbs, spices, and broth and bring to a boil.
5. Reduce the heat to low and simmer, partially covered for about 1 hour or until desired doneness.
6. Stir in the collard greens, salt and black pepper and cook for 4 minutes.
7. Stir in the lemon juice and remove from the heat.
8. Serve hot.

# Lentil & Quinoa Soup

**Yield:** 6 servings

**Preparation Time:** 15 minutes

**Cooking Time:** 40 minutes

**Total Time:** 55 minutes

**Ingredients:**

- 1 tablespoon coconut oil
- 3 carrots, peeled and chopped
- 2 celery stalks
- 1 onion, chopped
- 4 garlic cloves, minced
- 1½ teaspoons ground cumin
- 1 teaspoon red chili powder
- 4 cups tomatoes, chopped
- 1 cup red lentils, rinsed and drained
- ½ cup dried quinoa, rinsed and drained
- 5 cups homemade vegetable broth
- 2 cups fresh mustard greens, chopped

**Instructions:**

1. In a large soup pan, melt the coconut oil over medium heat and sauté the celery, onion and carrot for about 8-9 minutes.
2. Add the garlic and spices and sauté for about 1 minute.

3. Add the tomatoes, lentils, quinoa and broth and bring to
   a boil.
4. Reduce the heat to low and simmer, covered for about 20
   minutes.
5. Stir in mustard greens and simmer for about 4-5 minutes.
6. Stir in the salt and black pepper and remove from the
   heat.
7. Serve hot.

# Beans & Broccoli Soup

**Yield:** 4 servings

**Preparation Time:** 15 minutes

**Cooking Time:** 40 minutes

**Total Time:** 55 minutes

**Ingredients:**

- ¾ pound broccoli, chopped
- 1 tablespoon olive oil
- 1 onion, chopped
- 2 garlic cloves, minced
- 1 jalapeño pepper, seeded and chopped
- 2½ cups homemade vegetable broth
- 1½ cups cooked cannellini beans
- Sea salt and freshly ground black pepper, to taste

**Instructions:**

1. In a pan of the boiling water, add the broccoli and cook for about 3-4 minutes.
2. Drain the broccoli well.
3. In a large soup pan, heat the oil over medium heat and sauté onion for about 5 minutes.
4. Add the garlic and jalapeño pepper and sauté for about 1 minute.
5. Add the broth and beans and bring to a boil.

6.  Remove from the heat and set aside to cool slightly.

7.  In a blender, add the soup and broccoli in batches and pulse until smooth.

8.  Return the soup in the pan and cook for about 3-4 minutes.

9.  Season with the salt and black pepper and remove from the heat.

10. Serve hot.

# Dinner Recipes

## Mixed Mushrooms Stew

**Yield:** 4 servings

**Preparation Time:** 15 minutes

**Cooking Time:** 15 minutes

**Total Time:** 30 minutes

**Ingredients:**

- 2 tablespoons olive oil
- 2 onions, chopped
- 3 garlic cloves, minced
- ½ pound fresh button mushrooms, chopped
- ¼ pound fresh shiitake mushrooms, chopped
- ¼ pound fresh Portobello mushrooms, chopped
- Sea salt and freshly ground black pepper, to taste
- ¼ cup homemade vegetable broth
- ½ cup unsweetened coconut milk
- 2 tablespoons fresh parsley, chopped

**Instructions:**

1. In a large pan, heat the oil over medium heat and sauté the onion and garlic for 4-5 minutes.
2. Add the mushrooms, salt, and black pepper and cook for 4-5 minutes.

3.  Add the broth and coconut milk and bring to a gentle
    boil.
4.  Simmer for 4-5 minutes or until desired doneness.
5.  Stir in the parsley and remove from heat.
6.  Serve hot.

# Mixed Spicy Veggie Stew

**Yield:** 8 servings

**Preparation Time:** 20 minutes

**Cooking Time:** 35 minutes

**Total Time:** 55 minutes

**Ingredients:**

- 2 tablespoons coconut oil
- 1 large sweet onion, chopped
- 1 medium parsnip, peeled and chopped
- 3 tablespoons homemade tomato paste
- 2 large garlic cloves, minced
- ½ teaspoon ground cinnamon
- ½ teaspoon ground ginger
- 1 teaspoon ground cumin
- ¼ teaspoon cayenne pepper
- 2 medium carrots, peeled and chopped
- 2 medium purple potatoes, peeled and chopped
- 2 medium sweet potatoes, peeled and chopped
- 4 cups homemade vegetable broth
- 2 tablespoons fresh lemon juice
- 2 cups fresh kale, tough ribs removed and chopped
- ¼ cup fresh parsley leaves, chopped

**Instructions:**

1.  In a large soup pan, melt the coconut oil over medium-high heat and sauté the onion for about 5 minutes.

2.  Add the parsnip and sauté for about 3 minutes.

3.  Stir in the tomato paste, garlic, and spices and sauté for 2 minutes.

4.  Stir in carrots, potatoes, sweet potatoes, and broth and bring to a boil.

5.  Reduce the heat to medium-low and simmer, covered for about 20 minutes.

6.  Stir in the lemon juice and kale and simmer for 5 minutes.

7.  Serve with a topping of parsley.

# Herbed Mixed Veggie Stew

**Yield:** 8 servings

**Preparation Time:** 15 minutes

**Cooking Time:** 2¼ hours

**Total Time:** 2½ hours

**Ingredients:**

- 2 tablespoons coconut oil
- 1 medium yellow onions, chopped
- 2 cups celery, chopped
- ½ teaspoon garlic, minced
- 3 cups fresh kale, tough ribs removed and chopped
- ½ cup fresh mushroom, sliced
- 2½ cups tomatoes, chopped finely
- 1 teaspoon dried rosemary, crushed
- 1 teaspoon dried sage, crushed
- 1 teaspoon dried oregano, crushed
- Sea salt and freshly ground black pepper, to taste
- 2 cups homemade vegetable broth
- 3-4 cups alkaline water
- ¼ cup fresh parsley, chopped

**Instructions:**

1. In a large pan, melt the coconut oil over medium heat and sauté the onion, celery and garlic for about 5 minutes.

2.  Add the remaining all ingredients and stir to combine.

3.  Increase the heat to high and bring to a boil.

4.  Cook for about 10 minutes.

5.  Reduce the heat to medium and cook, covered for about 15 minutes.

6.  Uncover the pan and cook for about 15 minutes, stirring occasionally.

7.  Now, reduce the heat to low and simmer, covered for about 1½ hours.

8.  Serve hot with the garnishing of parsley.

# Tofu & Bell Pepper Stew

**Yield:** 6 servings

**Preparation Time:** 15 minutes

**Cooking Time:** 15 minutes

**Total Time:** 30 minutes

**Ingredients:**

- 2 tablespoons garlic
- 1 jalapeño pepper, seeded and chopped
- 1 (16-ounce) jar roasted red peppers, rinsed, drained and chopped
- 2 cups homemade vegetable broth
- 2 cups alkaline water
- 1 medium green bell pepper, seeded and sliced thinly
- 1 medium red bell pepper, seeded and sliced thinly
- 1 (16-ounce) package extra-firm tofu, drained and cubed
- 10 ounces frozen baby kale, thawed
- Sea salt and freshly ground black pepper, to taste

**Instructions:**

1. In a food processor, add the garlic, jalapeño pepper and roasted red peppers and pulse until smooth.
2. In a large pan, add the pepper puree, broth and water over medium-high heat and bring to a rolling boil.
3. Add the bell peppers and tofu and stir to combine.

4.  Reduce the heat to medium and cook for about 5 minutes.

5.  Stir in the kale and cook for about 5 minutes.

6.  Stir in the salt and black pepper and remove from the heat.

7.  Serve hot.

# Roasted Pumpkin Curry

**Yield:** 4 servings

**Preparation Time:** 15 minutes

**Cooking Time:** 35 minutes

**Total Time:** 50 minutes

**Ingredients:**

**For Roasted Pumpkin:**

- 1 medium sugar pumpkin, peeled and cubed
- Sea salt, to taste
- 1 teaspoon olive oil

**For Curry:**

- 1 teaspoon olive oil
- 1 onion, chopped
- 1 tablespoon fresh ginger root, peeled and minced
- 1 tablespoon garlic, minced
- 1 cup unsweetened coconut milk
- 2 cups vegetable broth
- 1 teaspoon ground cumin
- ½ teaspoon ground turmeric
- Sea salt and freshly ground black pepper, to taste
- 1 tablespoon fresh lime juice
- 2 tablespoons fresh parsley, chopped

## Instructions:

1. Preheat the oven to 400 degrees F. Line a large baking sheet with parchment paper.
2. In a large bowl, add all ingredients for the roasted pumpkin and toss to coat well.
3. Place pumpkin onto prepared baking sheet in a single layer.
4. Roast for about 20-25 minutes, flipping once halfway through.
5. Meanwhile, for curry: in a large pan, heat the oil over medium-high heat and sauté the onion for about 4-5 minutes.
6. Add the ginger and garlic and sauté for about 1 minute.
7. Add the coconut milk, broth, spices, salt, and black pepper and bring to a boil.
8. Reduce the heat to low and simmer for about 10 minutes.
9. Stir in the roasted pumpkin and simmer for 10 more minutes.
10. Serve hot with a garnish of parsley.

# Lentils, Veggies & Apple Curry

**Yield:** 6 servings

**Preparation Time:** 20 minutes

**Cooking Time:** 1½ hours

**Total Time:** 1 hour 50 minutes

**Ingredients:**

- 8 cups alkaline water
- ½ teaspoon ground turmeric
- 1 cup brown lentils
- 1 cup red lentil
- 1 tablespoon olive oil
- 1 large white onion, chopped
- 3 garlic cloves, minced
- 2 tomatoes, seeded and chopped
- ¼ teaspoon ground cloves
- 2 teaspoons ground cumin
- 2 carrots, peeled and chopped
- 2 potatoes, scrubbed and chopped
- 2 cups pumpkin, peeled, seeded and cubed into 1-inch size
- 1 granny smith apple, cored and chopped
- 2 cups fresh kale, tough ribs removed and chopped
- Sea salt and freshly ground black pepper, to taste

## Instructions:

1. In a large pan, add the water, turmeric and lentils over high heat and bring to a boil.
2. Reduce the heat to medium-low and simmer, covered for about 30 minutes.
3. Drain the lentils, reserving 2½ cups of the cooking liquid.
4. Meanwhile, in another large pan, heat the oil over medium heat and sauté the onion for about 2-3 minutes.
5. Add the garlic and sauté for about 1 minute.
6. Add the tomatoes and cook for about 5 minutes.
7. Stir in the spices and cook for about 1 minute.
8. Add the carrots, potatoes, pumpkin, cooked lentils and reserved cooking liquid and bring to a gentle boil.
9. Reduce the heat to medium-low and simmer, covered for about 40-45 minutes or until desired doneness of the vegetables.
10. Stir in apple and kale and simmer for about 15 minutes.
11. Stir in the salt and black pepper and remove from the heat.
12. Serve hot.

# Red Kidney Beans Curry

**Yield:** 6 servings

**Preparation Time:** 15 minutes

**Cooking Time:** 25 minutes

**Total Time:** 40 minutes

## Ingredients:

- 4 tablespoons olive oil
- 1 medium onion, chopped finely
- 2 garlic cloves, minced
- 2 tablespoons fresh ginger root, peeled and minced
- 1 teaspoon ground coriander
- 1 teaspoon ground cumin
- ½ teaspoon ground turmeric
- ¼ teaspoon cayenne pepper
- Sea salt and freshly ground black pepper, to taste
- 2 large plum tomatoes, chopped finely
- 3 cups cooked red kidney beans
- 2 cups alkaline water
- ¼ cup fresh parsley, chopped

## Instructions:

1. In a large pan, heat the oil over medium heat and sauté the onion, garlic, and ginger for about 6-8 minutes.

2. Stir in the spices and cook for about 1-2 minutes.

3. Stir in the tomatoes, kidney beans, and water and bring to a boil over high heat.

4. Reduce the heat to medium and simmer for 10-15 minutes or until desired thickness.

5. Serve hot with a garnish of parsley.

# Lentil & Carrot Chili

**Yield:** 8 servings

**Preparation Time:** 15 minutes

**Cooking Time:** 2 hours 40 minutes

**Total Time:** 2 hours 55 minutes

**Ingredients:**

- 2 teaspoons olive oil
- 1 large onion, chopped
- 3 medium carrots, peeled and chopped
- 4 celery stalks, chopped
- 2 garlic cloves, minced
- 1 jalapeño pepper, seeded and chopped
- ½ tablespoon dried thyme, crushed
- 1 tablespoon chipotle chili powder
- ½ tablespoon cayenne pepper
- 1½ tablespoons ground coriander
- 1½ tablespoons ground cumin
- 1 teaspoon ground turmeric
- Sea salt and freshly ground black pepper, to taste
- 1 pound red lentils, rinsed
- 8 cups homemade vegetable broth
- ½ cup scallion, chopped

**Instructions:**

1. In a large pan, heat the oil over medium heat and sauté the onion, carrot, and celery for about 5 minutes.
2. Add the garlic, jalapeño pepper, thyme, and spices and sauté for about 1 minute.
3. Add the lentils and broth and bring to a boil.
4. Reduce the heat to low and simmer, covered for about 2-2½ hours.
5. Remove from the heat and serve hot with a garnishing of scallion.

# Black Beans Chili

**Yield:** 5 servings

**Preparation Time:** 15 minutes

**Cooking Time:** 2 hours 5 minutes

**Total Time:** 2 hours 20 minutes

**Ingredients:**

- 2 tablespoons olive oil
- 1 onion, chopped
- 1 large green bell pepper, seeded and sliced
- 4 garlic cloves, minced
- 2 jalapeño peppers, sliced
- 1 teaspoon ground cumin
- 1 teaspoon cayenne pepper
- 1 tablespoon red chili powder
- 1 teaspoon paprika
- 2 cups tomatoes, chopped finely
- 4 cups cooked black beans
- 2 cups homemade vegetable broth
- Sea salt and freshly ground black pepper, to taste
- ¼ cup fresh parsley, chopped

**Instructions:**

1. In a large pan, heat the oil over medium-high heat and sauté the onion and bell peppers for 3-4 minutes.

2.  Add the garlic, jalapeño peppers and spices and sauté for about 1 minute.

3.  Add the remaining ingredients and bring to a boil.

4.  Reduce the heat to medium-low and simmer, covered for about 1½-2 hours.

5.  Season with the salt and black pepper and remove from the heat.

6.  Serve hot with the garnishing of parsley.

# Mixed Veggies Bake

**Yield:** 4 servings

**Preparation Time:** 15 minutes

**Cooking Time:** 20 minutes

**Total Time:** 35 minutes

**Ingredients:**

- 1 small zucchini, chopped
- 1 small summer squash, chopped
- 1 eggplant, cubed
- 1 red bell pepper, seeded and cubed
- 1 green bell peppers, seeded and cubed
- 1 onion, sliced thinly
- 1 tablespoon pure maple syrup
- 2 tablespoons olive oil
- Sea salt and freshly ground black pepper, to taste

**Instructions:**

1. Preheat the oven to 375 degrees F. Lightly, grease a large baking dish.
2. In a large bowl, add all the ingredients and mix well.
3. Transfer the vegetable mixture into the prepared baking dish.
4. Bake for about 15-20 minutes.
5. Remove from the oven and serve immediately.

# Veggie Ratatouille

**Yield:** 4 servings

**Preparation Time:** 20 minutes

**Cooking Time:** 45 minutes

**Total Time:** 1 hour 5 minutes

**Ingredients:**

- 6 ounces homemade tomato paste
- 3 tablespoons olive oil, divided
- ½ of onion, chopped
- 3 tablespoons garlic, minced
- Sea salt and freshly ground black pepper, to taste
- 1 zucchini, sliced into thin circles
- 1 yellow squash, sliced into circles thinly
- 1 eggplant, sliced into circles thinly
- 1 red bell pepper, seeded and sliced into circles thinly
- 1 yellow bell pepper, seeded and sliced into circles thinly
- 1 tablespoon fresh thyme leaves, minced
- 1 tablespoon fresh lemon juice

**Instructions:**

1. Preheat the oven to 375 degrees F.
2. In a bowl, add the tomato paste, 1 tablespoon of oil, onion, garlic, salt and black pepper and blend nicely.

3. In the bottom of a 10x10-inch baking dish, spread the tomato paste mixture evenly.

4. Arrange alternating vegetable slices, starting at the outer edge of the baking dish and working concentrically towards the center.

5. Drizzle the vegetables with the remaining oil and sprinkle with salt and black pepper, followed by the thyme.

6. Arrange a piece of parchment paper over the vegetables.

7. Bake for about 45 minutes.

8. Remove from the oven and serve hot.

# Quinoa with Veggies

**Yield:** 4 servings

**Preparation Time:** 15 minutes

**Cooking Time:** 26 minutes

**Total Time:** 41 minutes

**Ingredients:**

**For Roasted Mushrooms:**

- 2 cups small fresh Baby Bella mushrooms
- 1 tablespoon olive oil
- Sea salt, to taste

**For Quinoa:**

- 2 cups alkaline water
- 1 cup red quinoa, rinsed
- 2 tablespoons fresh parsley, chopped
- 1 garlic clove, minced
- 1 tablespoon olive oil
- 2 teaspoons fresh lemon juice
- Sea salt and freshly ground black pepper, to taste
- **For Broccoli:**
- 1 cup broccoli florets
- 2 tablespoons olive oil

**Instructions:**

1. Preheat the oven to 425 degrees F. Line a large rimmed baking sheet with parchment paper.
2. In a bowl, add the mushrooms, oil and salt and toss to coat well.
3. Arrange the mushroom onto the prepared baking sheet in a single layer.
4. Roast for about 15-18 minutes, tossing once halfway through.
5. Meanwhile, for quinoa: in a pan, add the water and quinoa over medium-high heat and bring to a boil.
6. Reduce the heat to low and simmer, covered for about 15-20 minutes or until all the liquid is absorbed.
7. Remove from the heat and set the pan aside, covered for about 5 minutes.
8. Uncover the pan and with a fork, fluff the quinoa.
9. Stir in the parsley, garlic, oil, lemon juice, salt and black pepper and set aside to cool completely.
10. Meanwhile, for broccoli: in a pan of the water, arrange a steamer basket and bring to a boil.
11. Place the broccoli florets in steamer basket and steam, covered for about 5-6 minutes.
12. Drain the broccoli florets well.
13. Transfer the broccoli florets into the bowl with quinoa and mushrooms and stir to combine.

14. Drizzle with the oil and serve immediately.

## Lentils with Kale

**Yield:** 6 servings

**Preparation Time:** 15 minutes

**Cooking Time:** 20 minutes

**Total Time:** 35 minutes

**Ingredients:**

- 1½ cups red lentils
- 1½ cups homemade vegetable broth
- 1½ tablespoons olive oil
- ½ cup onion, chopped
- 1 teaspoon fresh ginger, minced
- 2 garlic cloves, minced
- 1½ cups tomato, chopped
- 6 cups fresh kale, tough ribs removed and chopped
- Sea salt and ground black pepper, to taste

**Instructions:**

1. In a pan, add the broth and lentils over medium-high heat and bring to a boil.
2. Reduce the heat to and simmer, covered for about 20 minutes or until almost all the liquid is absorbed.

3.  Remove from the heat and set aside covered.

4.  Meanwhile, in a large skillet, heat the oil over medium heat and sauté the onion for about 5-6 minutes.

5.  Add the ginger and garlic and sauté for about 1 minute.

6.  Add the tomatoes and kale and cook for about 4-5 minutes.

7.  Stir in the lentils, salt and black pepper and remove from heat.

8.  Remove from the heat and serve hot.

# Lentils with Tomatoes

**Yield:** 4 servings

**Preparation Time:** 15 minutes

**Cooking Time:** 55 minutes

**Total Time:** 1 hour 10 minutes

**Ingredients:**

**For Tomato Puree:**

- 1 cup tomatoes, chopped
- 1 garlic clove, chopped
- 1 green chili, chopped
- ¼ cup alkaline water

**For Lentils:**

- 1 cup red lentils
- 3 cups alkaline water
- 1 tablespoon olive oil
- ½ of medium white onion, chopped
- ½ teaspoon ground cumin
- ½ teaspoon cayenne pepper
- ¼ teaspoon ground turmeric
- ¼ cup tomato, chopped
- ¼ cup fresh parsley leaves, chopped

**Instructions:**

1. For tomato paste in a blender, add all ingredients and pulse until a smooth puree forms. Set aside.
2. In a large pan, add 3 cups of water and lentils over high heat and bring to a boil.
3. Reduce the heat to medium-low and simmer, covered for about 15-20 minutes or until tender enough.
4. Drain the lentils well.
5. In a large skillet, heat the oil over medium heat and sauté the onion for about 6-7 minutes.
6. Add the spices and sauté for about 1 minute.
7. Add the tomato puree and cook, stirring for about 5-7 minutes.
8. Stir in the lentils and cook for about 4-5 minutes or until desired doneness.
9. Stir in the chopped tomato and immediately remove from heat.
10. Serve hot with the garnishing of parsley.

# Spicy Baked Beans

**Yield:** 4 servings

**Preparation Time:** 15 minutes

**Cooking Time:** 2 hours 5 minutes

**Total Time:** 2 hours 20 minutes

**Ingredients:**

- ½ pound dry red kidney beans, soaked overnight and drained
- 1¼ tablespoons olive oil
- 1 small yellow onion, chopped
- 4 garlic cloves, minced
- 1 teaspoon dried thyme, crushed
- ½ teaspoon ground cumin
- ½ teaspoon red pepper flakes, crushed
- ¼ teaspoon smoked paprika
- 1 tablespoon fresh lemon juice
- 1 cup homemade tomato sauce
- 1 cup homemade vegetable broth
- Sea salt and freshly ground black pepper, to taste

**Instructions:**

1. In a large pan of the boiling water, add the beans and bring to a boil.

2.  Reduce the heat to low and cook, covered for about 1 hour.

3.  Remove from the heat and drain the beans well.

4.  Preheat the oven to 325 degrees F.

5.  In a large oven-proof pan, heat the oil over medium heat and sauté the onion for about 4 minutes.

6.  Add the garlic, thyme and spices and sauté for about 1 minute.

7.  Stir in the cooked beans and remaining ingredients and immediately remove from the heat.

8.  Cover the pan and bake for about 1 hour.

9.  Remove from the oven and serve hot.

# Chickpeas with Pumpkin

**Yield:** 4 servings

**Preparation Time:** 20 minutes

**Cooking Time:** 35 minutes

**Total Time:** 55 minutes

**Ingredients:**

- 1 tablespoon olive oil
- 1 onion, chopped
- 2 garlic cloves, minced
- 1 green chili, seeded and chopped finely
- 1 teaspoon ground cumin
- ½ teaspoon ground coriander
- 1 teaspoon red chili powder
- 2 cups fresh tomatoes, chopped finely
- 2 pounds pumpkin, peeled and cubed
- 2 cups homemade vegetable broth
- 2 cups cooked chickpeas
- 2 tablespoons fresh lemon juice
- Sea salt and freshly ground black pepper, to taste
- 2 tablespoons fresh parsley leaves, chopped

**Instructions:**

1. In a large pan, heat oil over medium-high heat and sauté the onion for about 5-7 minutes.

2.  Add the garlic, green chili and spices and sauté for about
    1 minute.
3.  Add the tomatoes and cook for 2-3 minutes, crushing
    with the back of a spoon.
4.  Add pumpkin and cook for about 3-4 minutes, stirring
    occasionally.
5.  Add the broth and bring to a boil.
6.  Reduce the heat to low and simmer for about 10 minutes.
7.  Stir in the chickpeas and simmer for about 10 minutes.
8.  Stir in the lemon juice, salt, black pepper and remove
    from heat.
9.  Serve hot with the garnishing of parsley.

# Chickpeas with Kale

**Yield:** 6 servings

**Preparation Time:** 15 minutes

**Cooking Time:** 18 minutes

**Total Time:** 33 minutes

**Ingredients:**

- 2 tablespoons olive oil
- 1 medium onion, chopped
- 4 garlic cloves, minced
- 1 teaspoon dried thyme, crushed
- 1 teaspoon dried oregano, crushed
- ½ teaspoon paprika
- 1 cup tomato, chopped finely
- 2½ cups cooked chickpeas
- 4 cups fresh kale, tough ribs removed and chopped
- 2 tablespoons alkaline water
- 2 tablespoons fresh lemon juice
- Sea salt and freshly ground black pepper, to taste
- 3 tablespoons fresh basil, chopped

**Instructions:**

1. In a large skillet, heat the oil over medium heat and sauté the onion for about 8-9 minutes.

2.  Add the garlic, herbs and paprika and sauté for about 1 minute.
3.  Add the kale and water and cook for about 2-3 minutes.
4.  Add the tomatoes and chickpeas and cook for about 3-5 minutes.
5.  Stir in the lemon juice, salt and black pepper and remove from the heat.
6.  Serve hot with the garnishing of basil.

# Stuffed Cabbage Rolls

**Yield:** 4 servings

**Preparation Time:** 15 minutes

**Cooking Time:** 15 minutes

**Total Time:** 30 minutes

**Ingredients:**

**For Filling:**

- 1½ cups fresh button mushrooms, chopped
- 3¼ cups zucchini, chopped
- 1 cup red bell pepper, seeded and chopped
- 1 cup green bell pepper, seeded and chopped
- ½ teaspoon dried thyme, crushed
- ½ teaspoon dried marjoram, crushed
- ½ teaspoon dried basil, crushed
- Sea salt and freshly ground black pepper, to taste
- ½ cup homemade vegetable broth
- 2 teaspoons fresh lemon juice

**For Rolls:**

- 8 large cabbage leaves, rinsed
- 8 ounces homemade tomato sauce
- 3 tablespoons fresh parsley, chopped

## Instructions:

1. Preheat the oven to 400 degrees F. Lightly, grease a 13x9-inch casserole dish.
2. For filling: in a large pan, add all the ingredients except the lemon juice over medium heat and bring to a boil.
3. Reduce the heat to low and simmer, covered for about 5 minutes.
4. Remove from the heat and set aside for about 5 minutes.
5. Add the lemon juice and stir to combine.
6. Meanwhile, for rolls: in a large pan of the boiling water, add the cabbage leaves and boil for about 2-4 minutes.
7. Drain the cabbage leaves well.
8. Carefully, pat dry each cabbage leaf with paper towels.
9. Arrange the cabbage leaves onto a smooth surface.
10. With a knife, make a V shape cut in each leaf by cutting the thick vein.
11. Carefully, overlap cut ends of each leaf.
12. Place the filling mixture over each leaf evenly and fold in the sides.
13. Then, roll each leaf to seal the filling and then, secure each with toothpicks.
14. In the bottom of the prepared casserole dish, place 1/3 cup of the tomato sauce evenly.
15. Arrange the cabbage rolls over sauce in a single layer and top with remaining sauce evenly.

16. Cover the casserole dish and bake for about 15 minutes.

17. Remove from the oven and set aside, uncovered for about
    5 minutes.

18. Serve warm with the garnishing of the parsley.

# Green Beans & Mushroom Casserole

**Yield:** 6 servings

**Preparation Time:** 20 minutes

**Cooking Time:** 20 minutes

**Total Time:** 40 minutes

**Ingredients:**

**For Onion Slices:**

- ½ cup yellow onion, sliced very thinly
- ¼ cup almond flour
- 1/8 teaspoon garlic powder
- Sea salt and freshly ground black pepper, to taste

**For Casserole:**

- 1 pound fresh green beans, trimmed
- 1 tablespoon olive oil
- 8 ounces fresh cremini mushrooms, sliced
- ½ cup yellow onion, sliced thinly
- 1/8 teaspoon garlic powder
- Sea salt and freshly ground black pepper, to taste
- 1 teaspoon fresh thyme, chopped
- ½ cup homemade vegetable broth
- ½ cup coconut cream

**Instructions:**

1. Preheat the oven to 350 degrees F.
2. For onion slices: in a bowl, place all the ingredients and toss to coat well.
3. Arrange the onion slices onto a large baking sheet in a single layer and set aside.
4. For casserole: in a pan of salted boiling water, add the green beans and cook for about 5 minutes.
5. Drain the green beans and transfer them into a bowl of ice water.
6. Again, drain well and transfer them again into a large bowl. Set aside.
7. In a large skillet, heat oil over medium-high heat and sauté the mushrooms, onion, garlic powder, salt, and black pepper for about 2-3 minutes.
8. Stir in the thyme and broth and cook for about 3-5 minutes or until all the liquid is absorbed.
9. Remove from the heat and transfer the mushroom mixture into the bowl with the green beans.
10. Add the coconut cream and stir to combine well.
11. Transfer the mixture into a 10-inch casserole dish.
12. Place the casserole dish and baking sheet of onion slices into the oven.
13. Bake for about 15-17 minutes.

14. Remove the baking dish and sheet from the oven and let it cool for about 5 minutes before serving.

15. Top the casserole with the crispy onion slices evenly.

16. Cut into 6 equal-sized portions and serve.

# Wild Rice & Lentil Loaf

**Yield:** 8 servings

**Preparation Time:** 20 minutes

**Cooking Time:** 1 hour 50 minutes

**Total time:** 2 hours 10 minutes

**Ingredients:**

- 1¾ cups plus 2 tablespoons alkaline water, divided
- ½ cup wild rice
- ½ cup brown lentils
- Pinch of sea salt
- ½ teaspoon no-sodium Italian seasoning
- 1 medium yellow onion, chopped
- 1 celery stalk, chopped
- 6 cremini mushrooms, chopped
- 4 garlic cloves, minced
- ¾ cup rolled oats
- ½ cup pecans, chopped finely
- ¾ cup homemade tomato sauce
- ½ teaspoon red pepper flakes, crushed
- 1 teaspoon fresh rosemary, minced
- 2 teaspoons fresh thyme, minced

# Instructions:

1. In a pan, add 1¾ cups of water, rice, lentils, salt, and Italian seasoning and bring them to a boil over medium-high heat.
2. Reduce the heat to low and simmer covered for about 45 minutes.
3. Remove from the heat and set it aside, covered for at least 10 minutes.
4. Preheat the oven to 350 degrees F. Line a 9x5-inch loaf pan with parchment paper.
5. In a skillet, heat the remaining water over medium heat and sauté the onion, celery, mushrooms, and garlic for about 4-5 minutes.
6. Remove from the heat and let it cool slightly.
7. In a large mixing bowl, add the oats, pecans, tomato sauce, and fresh herbs and mix until well combined.
8. Combine the rice mixture and vegetable mixture with the oat mixture and mix well.
9. In a blender, add the mixture and pulse until a chunky mixture forms.
10. Transfer the mixture into the prepared loaf pan evenly.
11. With a piece of foil, cover the loaf pan and bake it for about 40 minutes.
12. Uncover and bake for about 15-20 minutes more or until the top becomes golden brown.

13. Remove it from the oven and set it aside for about 5-10 minutes before slicing.

14. Cut into desired sized slices and serve.

# Dessert Recipes

## Mixed Fruit Bowl

**Yield:** 10 servings

**Preparation Time:** 15 minutes

**Total Time:** 15 minutes

**Ingredients:**

**For Sauce:**

- ½ cup raw sunflower seeds
- 6 Medjool dates, pitted
- ½ cup unsweetened almond milk
- ½ teaspoon organic vanilla extract

**For Fruit Bowl:**

- 20 ounces fresh strawberries, hulled and sliced
- 1 pound fresh mango, peeled, pitted and cut into bite-sized pieces
- 1 pound fresh pineapples, peeled and cut into bite-sized pieces
- 2 bananas, peeled and sliced
- 2 cups fresh cherries, pitted
- 1 cup unsweetened coconut flakes, toasted
- 1 cup walnuts, toasted and chopped
- ¼ cup fresh mint leaves

**Instructions:**

1. For sauce: in a large bowl of alkaline water, soak the sunflower seeds overnight.
2. Drain the sunflower seeds well.
3. In a high-speed blender, add the sunflower seeds, dates, almond milk and vanilla extract and pulse until very smooth and creamy.
4. Transfer the sauce into a bowl and refrigerate until ready to serve.
5. For fruit bowl: in a serving bowl, add all the fruit into a bowl and mix.
6. Add the sauce and gentry, stir to combine.
7. Top with coconut and walnuts and serve with the garnishing of mint leaves.

# Cinnamon Peaches

**Yield:** 2 servings

**Preparation Time:** 15 minutes

**Cooking Time:** 6 minutes

**Total Time:** 21 minutes

**Ingredients:**

- 2 large peaches, halved and pitted
- ¼ cup chilled coconut cream
- 2-3 drops liquid stevia
- 1/8 teaspoon ground cinnamon
- 1 tablespoon walnuts, chopped

**Instructions:**

1. Preheat the grill to medium-high heat. Grease the grill grate.
2. Arrange the peach halves on the prepared grill, cut side down and cook for about 3-5 minutes per side.
3. Meanwhile, in a bowl, add the coconut cream and stevia and beat until fluffy.
4. Remove the peach halves from the grill and transfer onto serving plates.
5. Set aside to cool slightly.
6. Top each peach half with whipped coconut cream and sprinkle with cinnamon.

7. Garnish with walnuts and serve.

# Mixed Berries Granita

**Yield:** 4 servings

**Preparation Time:** 15 minutes

**Total Time:** 015 minutes

**Ingredients:**

- 1 cup fresh strawberries, hulled and sliced
- ½ cup fresh raspberries
- ½ cup fresh blackberries
- 1 tablespoon maple syrup
- 1 tablespoon fresh lemon juice
- 1 cup ice cubes, crushed
- 2 teaspoons fresh mint leaves

**Instructions:**

1. In a high-speed blender, add the berries, maple syrup, lemon juice, and ice cubes and pulse on high speed until smooth.
2. Transfer the berry mixture into an 8x8-inch baking dish and with the back of a spoon, spread in an even layer.
3. Freeze for at least 30 minutes.
4. Remove from the freezer and, with a fork, stir the granita completely.
5. Freeze for 2-3 hours, stirring every 30 minutes with a fork.

6. Garnish with mint leaves and serve.

# Chilled Mango Treat

**Yield:** 4 servings

**Preparation Time:** 10 minutes

**Total Time:** 10 minutes

**Ingredients:**

- 3 cups frozen mango, peeled, pitted, and chopped
- 1 tablespoon fresh mint leaves
- 2 tablespoons fresh lime juice
- ½ cup chilled water
- 2 tablespoons coconut, shredded

**Instructions:**

1. In a high-speed blender, add all the ingredients except coconut and pulse until smooth.
2. Transfer into serving bowls and serve immediately with the topping of coconut.

# Lemon Sorbet

**Yield:** 4 servings

**Preparation Time:** 10 minutes

**Cooking Time:** 1 minute

**Total Time:** 11 minutes

**Ingredients:**

- 2 tablespoons fresh lemon zest, grated
- ½ cup pure maple syrup
- 2 cups alkaline water
- 1½ cups fresh lemon juice
- 2 teaspoons fresh mint leaves

**Instructions:**

1. Freeze ice cream maker tub for about 24 hours before making this sorbet.
2. In a pan, add all of the ingredients except the lemon juice over medium heat and simmer for about 1 minute, stirring continuously.
3. Remove the pan from the heat and stir in the lemon juice.
4. Transfer the mixture into an airtight container and refrigerate for about 2 hours.
5. Now, transfer the mixture into an ice cream maker and process it according to the manufacturer's Instructions.

6.  Return the sorbet to the airtight container and freeze for about 2 hours.

7.  Serve with the garnishing of mint leaves.

# Mint & Coconut Mousse

**Yield:** 4 servings

**Preparation Time:** 15 minutes

**Total Time:** 15 minutes

**Ingredients:**

- 1½ cups raw coconut meat, chopped
- 1 tablespoon fresh mint leaves
- 1 tablespoon chia seeds
- 1¼ cups unsweetened almond milk
- 12 drops liquid stevia
- ¼ cup almond butter
- 1 teaspoon organic vanilla extract
- 3 tablespoons fresh raspberries

**Instructions:**

1. In a blender, add all ingredients except the raspberries and pulse until creamy and smooth.
2. Transfer into serving bowls and refrigerate to chill before serving.
3. Garnish with raspberries and serve.

# Chocolaty Beans & Oat Brownie

**Yield:** 12 servings

**Preparation Time:** 15 minutes

**Cooking Time:** 30 minutes

**Total Time:** 45 minutes

**Ingredients:**

- 2 cups cooked black beans
- 12 Medjool dates, pitted and chopped
- 2 tablespoons almond butter
- 2 tablespoons quick rolled oats
- 2 teaspoons organic vanilla extract
- ¼ cup cacao powder
- 1 tablespoon ground cinnamon

**Instructions:**

1. Preheat the oven to 350 degrees F. Line a large baking dish with parchment paper.
2. In a food processor, add all the ingredients except the cacao powder and cinnamon and pulse until well combined and smooth.
3. Transfer the mixture into a large bowl.
4. Add the cacao powder and cinnamon and stir to combine.

5.  Now, transfer the mixture into prepared baking dish
    evenly and with the back of a spatula, smooth the top
    surface.
6.  Bake for about 30 minutes.
7.  Remove from oven and place onto a wire rack to cool
    completely.
8.  With a sharp knife, cut into 12 equal-sized brownies and
    serve.

# Chickpeas Fudge

**Yield:** 12 servings

**Preparation Time:** 15 minutes

**Total Time:** 15 minutes

**Ingredients:**

- 2 cups cooked chickpeas
- 8 Medjool dates, pitted and chopped
- ½ cup almond butter
- ½ cup unsweetened almond milk
- 1 teaspoon organic vanilla extract
- 2 tablespoons cacao powder

**Instructions:**

1. Line a large baking dish with parchment paper.
2. In a food processor, add all the ingredients except cacao powder and pulse until well combined.
3. Transfer the mixture into a large bowl and stir in the cacao powder.
4. Transfer the mixture into the prepared baking dish, evenly spread. Smooth the surface with the back of a spatula.
5. Refrigerate for about 2 hours or until set completely.
6. Cut into desired sized squares and serve.

# Fruity Oatmeal Cookies

**Yield:** 18 servings

**Preparation Time:** 15 minutes

**Cooking Time:** 12 minutes

**Total Time:** 27 minutes

**Ingredients:**

- 2 teaspoons chia seeds
- ¼ cup warm alkaline water
- 2 cups quick oats, divided
- ½ teaspoon baking soda
- ½ teaspoon ground cinnamon
- ¼ teaspoon ground ginger
- ¼ cup raisins
- 1 large apple, peeled, cored and chopped
- 4 Medjool dates, pitted and chopped
- 1 teaspoon organic apple cider vinegar
- 2 tablespoons cold water

**Instructions:**

1. Preheat your oven to 375F. Line a large cookie sheet with a large greased parchment paper.
2. In a bowl, mix together warm water and chia seeds.
3. Set aside until thickened.

4. In a large food processor, add 1 cup of the oats and pulse until finely ground.

5. Transfer the ground oats in a large mixing bowl.

6. Add the remaining oats, baking soda, spices and raisins and mix well.

7. Now in the blender, add the remaining ingredients and pulse until smooth.

8. Transfer the apple mixture into the bowl with oat mixture and mix well.

9. Add the chia seeds mixture and stir to combine.

10. Spoon the mixture onto prepared cookie sheet in a single layer and with your finger, flatten each cookie slightly.

11. Bake for about 12 minutes or until golden brown.

12. Remove from oven and place the cookie sheet onto a wire rack to cool for about 5 minutes.

13. Now, invert the cookies onto the wire rack to cool before serving.

# Banana & Coconut Crumb

**Yield:** 2 servings

**Preparation Time:** 10 minutes

**Cooking Time:** 25 minutes

**Total Time:** 35 minutes

**Ingredients:**

- ¼ cup coconut, shredded
- 3 tablespoons coconut oil, melted
- 1 tablespoon fresh lemon juice
- ¼ teaspoon organic vanilla extract
- Pinch of ground cinnamon
- 2 medium bananas, peeled and sliced

**Instructions:**

1. Preheat the oven to 350 degrees F. Lightly, grease 2 ramekins.
2. In a bowl, add all ingredients except bananas and mix well.
3. In the bottom of the prepared ramekins, place the banana slices in and top with coconut mixture evenly.
4. Bake for about 25 minutes or until top becomes golden brown.
5. Remove from the oven and place the ramekins onto a wire rack to cool for about 5-10 minutes.

6.  Serve warm.

# Chapter 5: Conclusion

Ain't those recipes look luscious? Being on the Alkaline diet does not mean that the dieter must compromise on the flavors. There are tons of options that you can use to create a new healthy meal every time. And the recipes shared in this cookbook are just some delicious ideas that you can try at home. But you can always take things to the next level by adding more variety to the basic recipes, like adding a number of vegetables to the soup, mixing in fresh fruits to the salad and so on. Your diet can be as healthy as you want it to be and it can be as flavorsome as you desire, all its needs is a basic understanding of the dietary approach and the learning about the basic food items that can be used to create an entire men